THE LITTLE BOOK OF
PANDEMICS

50 of the world's most virulent plagues and infectious diseases

DR. PETER MOORE

THE LITTLE BOOK OF
PANDEMICS

50 of the world's most virulent plagues and infectious diseases

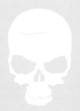

DR. PETER MOORE

Collins
An Imprint of HarperCollinsPublishers

FIRST U.S. EDITION

ISBN: 978-0-06-137421-0

Conceived and produced by
Elwin Street Limited
144 Liverpool Road
London N1 1LA
www.elwinstreet.com

Design: Alchemedia Design
Illustrations: Richard Burgess
Picture credits: All photographs © Science Photo Library

Printed and bound in China

Contents

Introduction

"A plague on both your houses!" shouts the fatally wounded Mercutio in Shakespeare's *Romeo and Juliet*, placing a desperate curse on the warring families. The word "plague" would have sent a ripple of fear down the spines of the people in his audiences, and the fact that they had no knowledge of the agent that swept invisibly across continents, devastating populations, and leaving families shattered and entire economies in tatters, only served to heighten the anxiety.

We have come a long way since Shakespeare's sixteenth century. We know about bacteria, viruses, and microscopic protozoa. We can watch the way that these tiny agents move into our bodies and damage our organs. We have a growing understanding of how our body mounts defensive strategies that fight off these invaders, and have built some clever chemicals that can help mount an assault on these bio-villains. In the middle of the twentieth century, as science was creating a new optimism, some serious commentators believed that the total eradication of nasty bacteria and viruses could be just a decade or so away. But it wasn't. Far from it. Our packed cities, linked by ever-faster systems of mass transport, are perfect breeding grounds for disease. Stand in a crowded train and, even if there is reasonably good ventilation, the air will have been in and out of ten or more people's lungs. The chemicals we have generated, such as antibiotics and anti-virals, are only around for a matter of months before the germ they are aimed at starts to learn how to duck and dodge. And, as overpopulation and the desire to exploit forests and jungles forces people to live side by side with other species, we provide the perfect environments for enabling germs that have previously only lived in animals to jump into humans.

From cholera to salmonella, Ebola to West Nile Virus, lives are being claimed every day. Some of these deaths are seemingly unavoidable consequences of natural disasters, others are exacerbated by war, poverty, or ignorance. Add to that the very real threat of biological weapons and terror attacks, and you have reason to sit up and think. After all, despite our technological advances we have only managed to drive one disease, smallpox, to the edge of extinction. Even then, the scientists wavered in indecision and decided not to destroy the last few vials, so laboratories around the world still contain stocks of this violent killer virus.

The good news is that while all of us will become infected with viruses, we normally do survive. Our bodies have a remarkably effective system for fighting disease, particularly one that they have experienced before. So, the list of diseases that follows, while alarming, does not mean that we are all doomed to die tonight. It does, however, point to the need for humble vigilance. We stand the best chance of keeping healthy by taking these invisible threats seriously.

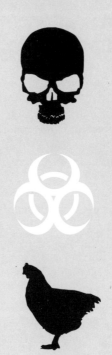

Part One:

Around and About – Community Diseases

Influenza

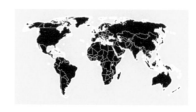

Agent: virus
Three types of influenza virus
(Family: *Orthomyxoviridae*)
First recorded: Hippocrates wrote about
a major epidemic in 412 B.C.E.
Region: global

Infectivity	
Severity of illness	
Likelihood of dying if ill	
Bio-weapon threat	

The influenza virus is a very simple biological particle in that it only contains eight genes, an instruction set so small that it cannot be described as being alive when it is floating freely in the air. However, like all viruses it comes to life when it invades a living cell and hijacks its biological machinery: in a matter of hours, one viral particle can dictate that the cell builds hundreds or thousands more new versions of itself.

Origins

For the recorded history of mankind, flu has normally caused only a low level of infection, but it occasionally breaks out and wreaks havoc. The good news about this virus is that most people become immune to it once they have encountered a particular strain. The bad news is that the virus evolves incredibly rapidly, and is constantly forming new strains. If a new strain is similar to one that has existed before, many people will fight it off, but on the occasions when there is a jump change—i.e. a rapid mutation in the virus—it can trigger a pandemic.

Symptoms and effects

If you think you have a "touch" of influenza, you probably don't. Flu hits hard. It will put you in bed for the best part of a week, and leave you weak for days after. As if that wasn't enough, if you get a bad bout you can end up suffering from depression for a further few days.

Historic outbreaks

Extreme outbreaks of flu occur about every 20 to 30 years. There was a massive pandemic in 1918 that killed somewhere around 40 million people; another severe outbreak killed between one and two million people in 1957; and yet another version killed some 700,000 people in 1968. Since then there has not been a major outbreak, but that means that the next one is getting closer.

Developments in treatment

In 1952 the World Health Organization set up a Global Influenza Surveillance Network, which consists of four key centers and 112 institutions located in 83 countries. The institutions collect and analyze samples, and ship any potential new strains to the centers. By monitoring which strains are circulating, experts make educated guesses about which pose the greatest threat in the near future. This information is sent to companies that manufacture vaccines, who then generate products that act against this specific threat. The vaccines offer a high level of protection, but the system only works as long as a new strain doesn't sneak up without warning. If a strain not covered by the vaccine starts to cause widespread disease, the vaccine is effectively useless.

A few anti-viral drugs are now making their way on to the market. Sadly, the rapidly evolving flu virus seems to be capable of side-stepping these with remarkable ease, taking the potency out of these newly hailed "wonder cures."

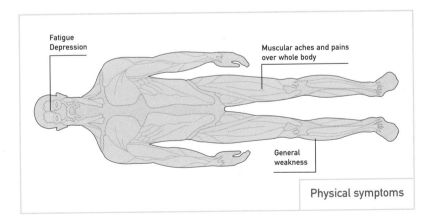

Fatigue
Depression

Muscular aches and pains over whole body

General weakness

Physical symptoms

H5N1 Bird Flu

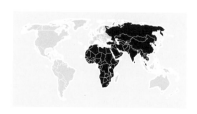

Agent: virus
H5N1 avian influenza A virus
(Family: *Orthomyxoviridae*)
First recorded: 2003
Region: mainly China, Asia and Africa

Infectivity	
Severity of illness	
Likelihood of dying if ill	
Bio-weapon threat	

The previous entry shows just how devastating a new version of influenza can be. No surprise, then, that people who know the history of previous flu pandemics are starting to get alarmed that a version of flu that has only ever attacked birds has evolved so that it can also infect humans.

The flu virus is microscopically small and covered with spikes, which are two different types of protein: the "H" protein helps the virus break into cells, while the "N" protein enables it to get out again. In the influenza range of viruses there are 12 different basic H proteins and nine known N types; however, the viruses constantly generate minor variations of each protein, which can cause major changes in its function. While viruses with H1N1, H1N2, and H3N2 frequently attack humans, those with the other protein spikes normally leave us alone. H5N1 strains normally limit their activity to birds, but this one has evolved so that it can jump to people.

Origins

The first victim we know of died in 2003; another person from the same family then became ill. Both lived in Hong Kong, but appear to have picked up the bug while visiting mainland China. It is quite possible that people had been dying of this virus for months, but that the deaths were either not investigated, or not reported to the rest of the world. Scientific reports show that this virus was certainly in some Chinese bird flocks as early as 1996.

The virus probably managed to jump species because so many people in rural China live so close to their animals. Sharing a living space with poultry and pigs is a great way of coming into contact with their excrement and with all the bugs lurking in it. This constant exposure means that if a virus happens to develop the potential to get into a human, it has a good chance of finding an opportunity to do so.

Symptoms and effects

The first symptoms are like those of any other flu bug: headache, fever, aching muscles, itching eyes, and a sore throat. If it follows the pattern of previous flu viruses that have jumped the species gap, it will also cause pneumonia in a large number of

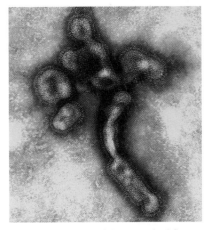

Above Human strain of the H5N1 bird flu virus, isolated during the 2003 outbreak.

people. This occurs because the virus damages the lining of the lungs, allowing fluid to escape into the air space. This prevents oxygen and carbon dioxide from moving in and out of the body, so the person will gradually turn blue and breathless. On top of this, the fluid is a perfect breeding ground for bacteria, so you end up with a potentially lethal mixture of diseases.

At the beginning of 2006 there were only a few reports suggesting that the virus could pass from human to human, but none of these had been confirmed. Human-to-human infection poses the biggest problem. If the disease can only move to humans from animals, there is the possibility of containing it by avoiding, or, if necessary, culling, the animals. However, if it ever starts moving between people, the disease becomes very difficult to control.

Region of operation

While this virus started life in China, it has now spread far and wide, carried by a mixture of a cavalier attitude to agricultural trade and the unstoppable migration of wild birds. Over a two-year period it spread across Eastern Asia, through Russia, and down into Africa. Migrating birds then moved it northwards from Africa into Europe.

Developments in treatment

As with all viral diseases there are very few treatment options, and the few drugs available have a poor track record in the people who have received them. On top of this, the virus seems to be able to evolve very rapidly to defeat the therapy. Vaccination is a hope, but the problem here is that the vaccine needs to be specifically targeted at an individual strain of virus. Only when the virus mutates to a human-to-human form will the pharmaceutical companies be able to start building the vaccine, and it will take months for it to become available. That could be too late for many people.

Headache
Fever
Itching eyes
Sore throat
Lung damage and pneumonia

Physical symptoms

Potential threat to civilization

H5N1 poses a distinct threat to civilization as we know it, not so much in the numbers of people who might be killed—though that could be bad enough—but more because of the probable reactions to any pandemic. In the short term governments could place severe restrictions on travel, which would impact food and energy supplies, and bring trade and commerce to a temporary halt. The resulting shortages could trigger widespread disruption and civil disorder—it's not a happy prospect. On the other hand, this version of the virus may never learn how to trouble humans in a big way, and the hype will die away with the disease.

MRSA

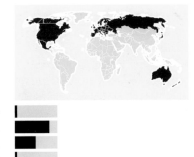

Agent: bacterium
Methicillin-resistant *Staphylococcus aureus*
First recorded: 1961
Region: Developed countries

Infectivity	
Severity of illness	
Likelihood of dying if ill	
Bio-weapon threat	

MRSA—or methicillin-resistant *Staphylococcus aureus*—is a bacterium that makes those in the know shudder a little. Not so much because it is a terrifying killer—it can be pretty harmless—but more because it stands as a glaring reminder that we have not won the war against bacteria. As its name suggests, MRSA is a type of bacteria that can cause serious harm, even death, but is resistant to methicillin, one of the most potent antibiotics in the medical armory.

Origins

In the late 1920s, London-based doctor Alexander Fleming spotted that a strain of mold growing in a laboratory Petri dish seemed to be capable of killing bacteria if they came too close. The end result of this observation was that we now have antibiotics—a class of drugs that kill bacterial cells, but don't kill animal cells. This miraculous breakthrough has transformed medicine for people wealthy enough to use antibiotics. A simple scratch that could have killed you by allowing bacteria to break into the body is now of little concern. If you do get an infection, a few days of tablets will solve the problem.

Bacteria, however, haven't just rolled over and admitted defeat. The fact that they have performed spectacularly well on the planet for millions of years stems from their ability to adapt to new challenges, and normally to come out on top. In the case of antibiotics, it was only a matter of months before Fleming found that some bacteria rapidly learned how to evade his early versions of the chemical. At first, the solution was simple: invent another antibiotic, and challenge the adapted bacteria with that. The new antibiotic

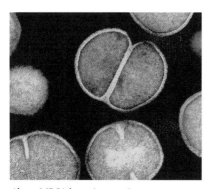

Above MRSA bacteria are resistant to most antibiotics, meaning they are very hard to get rid of and control.

works for a while, but after a few weeks or months, strains of bacteria appear that can now cope not only with this newcomer, but with the old one as well.

In the 1960s, a strain of bacteria called *Staphylococcus aureus* started to learn how to evade the killing power of the antibiotic methicillin. This antibiotic is only used to tackle bacteria that are already resistant to most other drugs. *S. aureus* is extremely common in the open environment and lives in the noses and skin of most people without causing any problems, but occasionally it gets out of control and sets up an infection. If these infections cannot be controlled, a person's life is in danger. Now that many of these bacteria are resistant to antibiotics, fighting them can be a lot harder.

Symptoms and effects

You can be colonized with MRSA for years and not know it, but if the bugs start multiplying rapidly and set up an infection, you will develop hot red patches at the site of the growing bacteria, and the area will also swell and become tender. The bacteria most commonly colonize the nostrils, but the respiratory tract, open wounds, and urinary tracts are also potential sites of infection. People with compromised immune systems who contract an infection are also at great risk of contracting a secondary infection.

Region of operation

The myth is that MRSA is something you catch only in hospitals. However, there is actually plenty of it out in the wider community, and many people who appear to catch it while they are lying in a hospital bed probably brought it with them. The infection flared up because they were ill—that's why they were in hospital in the first place. The problem with being ill is that your defenses are weakened and you are therefore less capable of controlling bacteria that may have found a comfortable home in your nostril or some crevice of the skin.

This isn't the full story, though. Some people do pick up the disease while in hospital. This is partly because resistant bacteria occur where antibiotics are used, and there are more antibiotics being used in hospitals than anywhere else in the community. Hospitals are therefore breeding grounds for these specialist bacteria. The task, then, is to make it hard for bugs to jump from one patient to the next, and the simplest and most effective measure here is for staff and visitors to wash their hands before going to see a patient. MRSA doesn't travel well—washing your hands with a germ-killing soap can easily spoil its fun.

Developments in treatment

Becoming infected with MRSA is not a death sentence. Using a cocktail of antibiotics over a period of time can often clear the infection. At the same time, the race is on to find alternatives to antibiotics, but finding new ways of damaging bacterial cells while leaving our own cells healthy has not been easy.

An alternative might be to use a range of viruses that infect and destroy bacteria. Researchers in the former Soviet Union spent many years developing their ability to use these "bacteriophage," but with the breakdown of the Union this work ground to a halt. Now, however, a few pharmaceutical companies are starting to take them seriously.

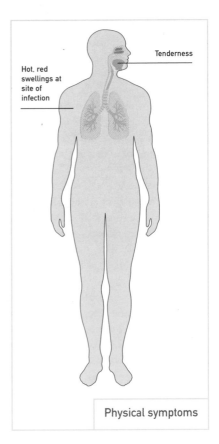

Tenderness

Hot, red swellings at site of infection

Physical symptoms

Chicken Pox

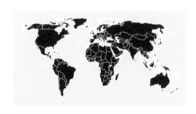

Agent: virus
Varicella-zoster virus
(Family: *Herpesviridae*)
First recorded: ancient China and ancient Greece
Region: global

Infectivity	
Severity of illness	
Likelihood of dying if ill	
Bio-weapon threat	

Chicken pox is one of the most contagious diseases known to man. Around 95 percent of people will have been infected with it by the time they reach adulthood. The good news is that almost all of them will survive the attack.

Varicella is part of the herpes virus family, which consists of around 100 viruses—eight of which are known to cause diseases that affect humans.

Symptoms and effects

For the first few days after becoming infected, a person has no symptoms. Then, between 10 and 21 days later, a red, itchy rash starts to appear. The first spots show up on the chest and back, then new pimples rapidly appear on most of the body. The ones on the face, nose, mouth, and ears can be particularly irritating, as can any that develop on the genitals.

The spots come out in bouts over two to four days. A mildly affected person can get away with fewer than ten; a severely affected person will have thousands. Anyone who has a major outbreak of spots is also very likely to run a high fever. Over the following days the spots develop into fluid-filled blisters that then burst and dry over. Eventually, the dry scabs fall off, taking with them the last viruses that are locked into the scabs.

One of the problems with chicken pox is that a person can pass on the disease for two days before the first spots show. In fact, it is at its most contagious the day before the spots appear.

Historic outbreaks

One good thing about chicken pox is that very few people get it twice, as the first infection triggers a life-long immunity to the disease. Another good thing comes, paradoxically, from the fact that it is highly contagious. Ninety percent of children living in a household where someone has chicken pox will catch it, and 20 percent of children whose playmates have it will get the disease. As a consequence, it infects the majority of people by the age of eight. This means that, while it can sweep through a playgroup or infant school, it is unlikely to cause a major pandemic as so many people are immune to the disease.

Developments in treatment

Since 1995, some doctors have been giving a vaccine to children who are over 12 months old and have not already had the disease. It has a high track record in preventing people from getting chicken pox, and in the United States there is an active drive to encourage everyone to take the vaccine. Other countries are holding back from this, considering that the cost of the vaccination program is not justified as the disease seldom produces long-term damage.

Another option is to give a person a dose of *varicella-zoster* immune globulin. This can specifically boost a person's ability to fight the disease, but the protection only lasts for three weeks; after this, the globulin is removed from the body and the protective effect goes with it.

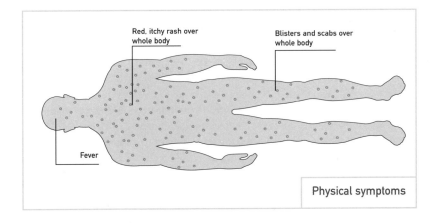

Red, itchy rash over whole body

Blisters and scabs over whole body

Fever

Physical symptoms

Anthrax

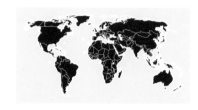

Agent: bacterium
Bacillus anthracis
First recorded: 1500 B.C.E. in Egypt
Region: Global, but particularly South
and Central America, Southern and
Eastern Europe, Asia, Africa, the
Caribbean, and the Middle East

Infectivity	
Severity of illness	
Likelihood of dying if ill	
Bio-weapon threat	

An outbreak of boils in ancient Egypt is probably the first recorded incidence of anthrax, and it has continued to cause social and economic damage ever since. The bacterium survives in soil and is easily picked up by grazing animals, then passed on to humans who work with them or eat their meat. The bacteria are also quite happy to skip the intermediary and jump straight to humans, either through a cut in the skin or through the lungs as we breathe.

Symptoms and effects

Whether you have a mild attack or run the risk of being killed depends largely on how the bacteria get in. In about 95 percent of cases, anthrax gets into people through their skin. The first a victim knows of it is when he or she starts to itch and has a spot that looks much like an insect bite. Within a couple of days, the spot develops into a painless ulcer that is about 0.4–1.2 inches (1–3 cm) wide, and has a dark area in the middle where the skin is dead or dying. If left untreated, this infection will kill one in five people.

Contracting the disease by eating contaminated meat causes nausea. The person then loses their appetite, starts vomiting, and has a fever. If untreated, this moves on to diarrhea and vomiting blood. Between 25 and 60 percent die.

Getting the disease by inhaling the agent is normally fatal within a few days. The symptoms start like a common cold, but soon move on to severe breathing difficulties and shock—not nice.

Developments in treatment

Antibiotics can help to fight the milder forms of the illness, and vaccination is a possible option for people who encounter the bacteria at work. That said, the pace at which the disease develops means that there is still little that can be done to save someone with the inhaled form of the disease.

Used as a weapon

While anthrax is a constant threat to many agricultural communities around the world, it made world headlines in 2001. Just under a month after the 9/11 attack on the World Trade Center, 63-year-old Robert Stevens died in a hospital in Atlantis, Florida, two days after developing breathing problems and a high fever. It turned out that he had inhaled anthrax spores while in his office. He worked for American Media, a Florida-based company that owned a tabloid newspaper that had published insulting articles about Osama bin Laden. Over the next few weeks, spores and infected people showed up in only a few places, but the resultant panic affected the entire United States.

The particular strain of anthrax used was not naturally occuring; it had been artificially modified and mixed with chemicals so that it floated in the air for longer than natural anthrax, maximizing the chances of it being inhaled. In technical speak, it had been "weaponized," and the best guess is that it had been stolen from the U.S. army. The perpetrator has never been found.

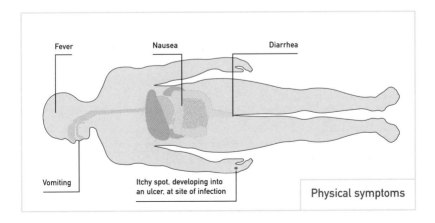

Fever

Nausea

Diarrhea

Vomiting

Itchy spot, developing into an ulcer, at site of infection

Physical symptoms

Bacterial Meningitis

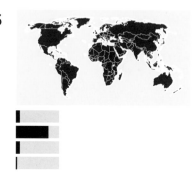

Agent: bacterium
Many different bacteria
First recorded: Middle Ages (1300s)
Region: global

Infectivity	
Severity of illness	
Likelihood of dying if ill	
Bio-weapon threat	

Your brain and spinal cord are encased inside protective bone and wrapped in the meninges, a tough three-layered membrane. The layers are lubricated with some of the cerebrospinal fluid that washes over the brain. Meningitis occurs when this fluid or the membranes become infected. The disease can become more complicated if the infection also becomes established in the person's bloodstream, as they now have septicemia (diseased blood) as well.

Origins
There are a few viruses that occasionally infect the meninges, but these seldom cause any severe damage. Occasionally, fungal infections can attack the meninges, but bacterial infections are the ones to worry about and can be caused by one of 50 or more different bugs. The most common causes are infections of either meningococcal or pneumococcal bacteria, but *Haemophilus influenzae b* (Hib), *Group B Streptococcal bacteria, Escherichia coli, Listeria*, and the bacteria that cause tuberculosis can all set up shop in the meninges. They all carry different scales of risk and severity of disease, but all can kill or leave people permanently disabled.

Symptoms and effects
The classic signs to look for are a combination of fever, headache, vomiting, stiff neck, drowsiness, and an inability to cope with bright lights. However, these symptoms are common to many other diseases. A more conclusive symptom develops in some people: a rash of red spots that look a bit like pin-pricks and then spread out to become larger spots, purple bruises, or blood

blisters. These marks are distinctive because if you press a glass against them they don't fade. This is because blood has broken out of the vessels that normally contain it, so when you press the blood cannot escape. If you see this effect, you need immediate medical help.

Historic outbreaks

Pandemics of meningitis occur about every eight to ten years in areas of sub-Saharan Africa. In 1996, the W.H.O. recorded almost 190,000 cases in Burkina Faso, Chad, Mali, Niger, and Nigeria. The outbreak was so severe that it paralyzed the routine health-care systems in these countries and exhausted the international stocks of vaccine. Partly as a response to this, an International Coordinating Group (I.C.G.) for Vaccine Provision for Epidemic Meningitis Control was established in 1997.

Developments in treatment

Treating bacterial meningitis is complicated by the fact that so many bacteria can resist different antibiotics. Ideally, doctors need to work out exactly which type of bacteria is present, then find a set of antibiotics that will kill them. This can, however, take a couple of days or longer, so in practice doctors take an educated guess about which antibiotics to use at first, then switch treatment if tests show that other antibiotics are more likely to wipe out the microbes.

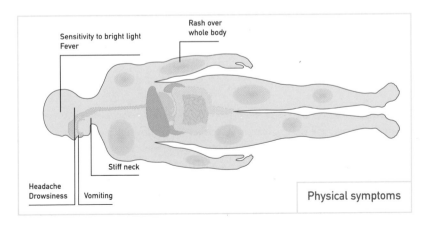

Sensitivity to bright light
Fever

Rash over whole body

Stiff neck

Headache
Drowsiness

Vomiting

Physical symptoms

Leprosy

Agent: bacterium
Mycobacterium leprae
First recorded: 1500s B.C.E.
Region: developing world

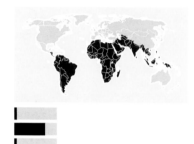

Infectivity	
Severity of illness	
Likelihood of dying if ill	
Bio-weapon threat	

The bacterium that causes leprosy is a close cousin of the one that causes tuberculosis, and both diseases are proving hard to eradicate. When discussing leprosy, we first need to dispel a few myths. It is not a flesh-eating condition, and it is not easy to pass it from one person to another: shaking hands with someone who has the disease will not give you leprosy. It is also easy to control with modern drugs—the reason why there is so much leprosy still about is largely because those who suffer are poor and can't afford the medication.

Origins

Writings in the sixteenth century B.C.E. show that Egyptians thought the disease came from bathing in the Nile. Records show that leprosy was probably a relatively common disease in India in the fifteenth century B.C.E., and in Japan in the tenth century B.C.E., and the best guess is that it came to Western Europe and beyond via Egypt. In the second century C.E., the Greek/Roman doctor Galen believed that leprosy was caused by people having a poor diet.

Symptoms and effects

If left untreated, the disease leaves victims without the ability to feel pain in various parts of their body, such as the toes and fingers. The loss of the warning signal for pain makes it all too easy for these areas to become damaged. This damage may be so severe that the person loses digits or limbs, or it may simply enable other bacteria to come on board and trigger further disease. Either way, if the disease is left untreated, infected people can soon be in real difficulty.

Region of operation

Rates of infection are beginning to fall. In 2002, three-quarters of a million new cases of leprosy were reported to the W.H.O., but this had dropped to just over 400,000 by 2004. Most cases show up in developing nations, with Brazil, Madagascar, Mozambique, Tanzania, and Nepal accounting for over 90 percent of the count. Don't get complacent in developing countries, though: there are about 100 new cases each year in the United States. Add together all the people who either have the disease currently, or who are still suffering from its side effects, and you reach a total of between one and two million worldwide.

Developments in treatment

In the 1950s, doctors started to give sufferers a drug called dapsone. At first, this had powerful effects in killing the bacteria. It didn't restore any functions that victims had lost, but it did prevent them from getting worse. Dapsone, however, soon went the way of so many drug therapies, and it was only a few years before drug-resistant strains of the bacteria emerged. Over the 1970s and 1980s, two other drugs were developed and treatment now involves giving people all three. This multi-drug therapy hits the bug so hard that it has no chance of surviving long enough to adapt. Within a couple of days a person will no longer be able to pass the disease on, but it will take six to twelve months of regular treatment for the bacteria to be driven out of a sufferer's body.

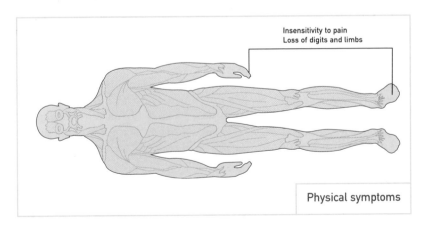

Insensitivity to pain
Loss of digits and limbs

Physical symptoms

Smallpox

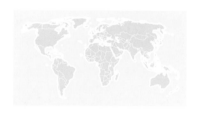

Agent: virus
Variola
(Family: *Orthopoxvirus*)
First recorded: 1157 B.C.E. on the
mummified body of Ramses V of Egypt
Region: a few laboratory freezers

Infectivity	
Severity of illness	
Likelihood of dying if ill	
Bio-weapon threat	

Smallpox probably originated in India or Egypt over 3,000 years ago. As late as the 1950s, some 150 years after English doctor Edward Jenner introduced the first vaccine for the disease, an estimated 50 million cases of the disease occurred every year, and one in three infected people died.

A massive eradication campaign started in 1967, with the last natural case of the disease being in Somalia in 1977. We had driven smallpox off the face of the earth. Well, almost. Realizing that there were no more viruses in the wild that could infect people, academic scientists then hesitated over the task of destroying the few remaining stocks that they held in two sets of laboratory freezers—one in the Soviet Union, the other in the U.S.A. Three times they passed global destruction dates without casting the remnant into incinerators.

Then the Soviet Union fell apart and so did any ability to control their scientists and the laboratory stocks. No one really knows what happened to the smallpox-virus-containing vials, as the scientists left former Soviet-bloc countries in search of work. The fear that some are now held by people who may have less than friendly designs on Western nations has been enough to persuade Western scientists to hang tenaciously on to their stocks. The claim is that this retention is not so that the West could revenge any deliberate terror-raising release of smallpox in a biological form of "tit for tat," but so that Western scientists can research the infective and killing power of the disease, and therefore be better prepared for combat.

Smallpox could be seen as the disease that got away; but hopefully it will not become the come-back kid.

Symptoms and effects

Smallpox is serious. There are many different types and sub-types, but "variola major smallpox" accounted for nine out of ten infections. "Variola modified smallpox" occurred occasionally in people who had been vaccinated, while "variola flat" and "variola hemorrhagic smallpox" were both very severe, but thankfully extremely rare.

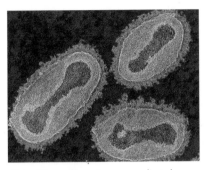

Above The smallpox virus was eradicated thanks to a global vaccination program in the 1970s, but still exists in some laboratories for research purposes.

Somewhere between 7 and 17 days after meeting the virus, victims start to develop a fever, feel generally ill, and develop a headache. They are normally too sick to carry on normal daily activities, and have to retire to bed. They probably don't realize they have the disease, but can already pass it on to other people.

After a couple of days, a rash starts to appear, initially as small spots on the tongue and in the mouth. The spots grow and break open into sores that release millions of new viral particles. These can be coughed into the air or swallowed. Either through airborne droplets or feces, the virus moves off to find other hosts.

The virus not only leaves the body, it also spreads through it. Spots start appearing all over the body, developing into sores that fill with thick, opaque fluid. A highly characteristic feature of the disease is that these spots normally develop a dip in the middle and look much like a belly button. The person's temperature soars. For the next five days, the sores become hard to the touch, as if there were a pellet inside each one. If you survive, they begin to scab over and fall off, leaving marks on the skin that eventually become pitted scars. It is only when the last scab drops off and is carefully swept away that you cease to be infectious.

Developments in treatment

Smallpox was the first disease to be tackled by vaccination, as Edward Jenner exposed people to cowpox. The virus causing this disease was a close cousin to smallpox, and an infection with this virus was safe, but triggered immunity to all *variola* viruses. We still remember that this form of medical miracle has its origins in cows due to the name of the procedure—*vacca* is Latin for cow.

Used as a weapon

If you are in doubt as to whether smallpox could be used as a weapon, ask yourself a simple question: why, post 9/11, have the U.S. authorities stockpiled enough smallpox vaccine to inoculate their entire population? Answer: they fear that someone may get hold of a vial of the virus and deliberately release it. The U.S. intelligence services believe that it is a threat that needs to be taken seriously.

The virus would be such an effective weapon because so many people in the world are now not immunized against the disease. Because it has been driven to extinction, there seemed no point in spending vast fortunes keeping up our immunity to a dead disease. People living in countries that don't have similar stockpiles can only hope that no one resurrects it.

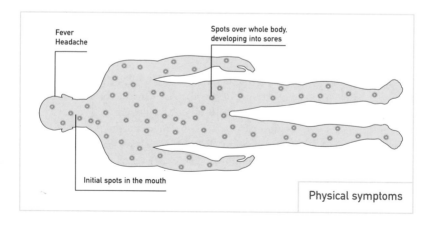

Fever
Headache

Spots over whole body, developing into sores

Initial spots in the mouth

Physical symptoms

Ebola

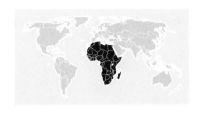

Agent: *Filoviridae* virus
Ebola-Zaire, Ebola-Sudan, Ebola-Ivory
Coast, and Ebola-Reston
First recorded: 1976
Region: mainly Africa

Infectivity	
Severity of illness	
Likelihood of dying if ill	
Bio-weapon threat	

Even within the nightmare class of viruses, Ebola stands in a class of its own. Its ability to appear unannounced and wreak havoc for a few months before disappearing from view gives it a reputation of unpredictable menace. Everyone knows that it hasn't gone for good: it's just biding its time, waiting for another opportunity.

Origins

The virus was first recorded in 1976 in Zaire (now known as the Democratic Republic of Congo), when 318 people living on the banks of the river Ebola and in the surrounding area became ill, 280 of whom died. In the same year, 284 people became ill in Sudan, 151 of whom died. By 2004, a total of 1,848 people had been recorded as having caught the disease, with 1,287 of these not surviving the experience—a high kill rate. The numbers are not huge, but thankfully it has so far only broken out in fairly dispersed rural populations.

As well as the Democratic Republic of Congo and Sudan, cases of Ebola have sprung up in Uganda, Gabon, and Ivory Coast. It is probably passed to humans from animals but, despite considerable research, no one yet knows for sure where it hides between outbreaks. The finger of suspicion points to monkeys, and it probably moves into humans when someone eats an infected monkey.

Once in a human, it is transmitted between people as they come into contact with infected blood or other bodily fluids, which means that anyone caring for an infected person is at particular risk. Re-using needles or pushing

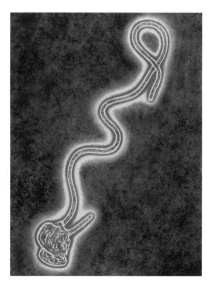

Above Ebola is part of the group of filoviruses, so called because of the thin and long shape of the viruses.

infected needles into multi-dose bottles of medicine are alternative ways of spreading it around. So too is any form of physical contact with a person who has died of the disease, which means that many ritual burial practices have to be curtailed if an outbreak is going to be contained.

Symptoms and effects

Ebola hemorrhagic fever kills between 50 and 90 percent of people who become infected, and the mode of death is unpleasant. Once infected, people start to get a fever within two to 21 days. They suddenly become very weak, and have muscle, joint, or abdominal pains, headache, sore throat, nausea, and exhaustion. So far, it could be one of many far more common diseases—these early symptoms are easily mistaken for malaria, typhoid fever, dysentery, influenza, or various bacterial infections. But then the bleeding starts. Their eyes start to turn red as blood seeps from damaged blood vessels, red spots appear due to bleeding under the skin, they cough and vomit blood-red foam as their lungs and guts start to weaken, and inside the body the virus is causing severe organ damage, especially to the kidneys, liver, and spleen. Bloody diarrhea adds to the horror. By the second week of infection, either the fever will lessen, or the patient will die from organ failure. The amount of time from the onset of symptoms to death is usually between seven and fourteen days.

As scientists have traced Ebola's destructive path, they have determined that there are currently four distinct sub-types of the disease. They each cause a similar spectrum of symptoms, but the chance of dying from them is different. Ebola-Zaire is the main one to avoid, as it kills about 90 percent of those who become clinically ill. Ebola-Sudan kills "only" 50 percent. Not many people have been infected with Ebola-Ivory Coast, but all have survived. Ebola-Reston is a potential worry. So far it has only infected monkeys, but it has raised huge concerns as outbreaks of the disease have occurred in research laboratories in the United States and Italy. It would, after all, only take a minor chance mutation for this virus to learn how to leap into humans.

Developments in treatment

There is no treatment for Ebola, other than to try to keep the patient as comfortable as possible—making sure their oxygen and blood levels are maintained and treating them for any secondary infections, and hope that their own immune system activates in time. One of the few things that is known about the disease is that those who die show little sign that the immune system recognized that the virus was on board. How such a destructive virus sneaks in unnoticed is a matter of considerable scientific interest.

Used as a weapon

Currently, there is little fear that Ebola will be used as a weapon, but there were Cold War rumors that Soviet scientists were trying to marry the killing power of Ebola with the infective power of smallpox. Let's hope that either the rumors were untrue, or that they failed.

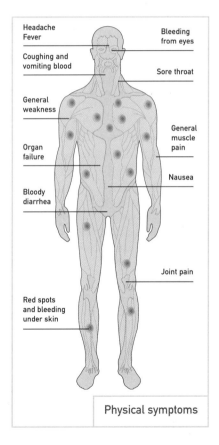

Physical symptoms

Headache
Fever

Coughing and vomiting blood

General weakness

Organ failure

Bloody diarrhea

Red spots and bleeding under skin

Bleeding from eyes

Sore throat

General muscle pain

Nausea

Joint pain

Group A Streptococci

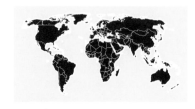

Agent: bacterium
Streptococcus pyogenes
First recorded: 1874
Region: global

Infectivity	▉▉
Severity of illness	▉
Likelihood of dying if ill	▏
Bio-weapon threat	▏

Take the name to pieces and it doesn't seem so daunting: *streptos* is Greek for chain and *coccos* means grain or berry. Down a microscope, that is all you see—chains of small balls—but mass these together and they can kill.

Origins

Group A *streptococci* are powerful because they are versatile. They have a number of modes of attack and can set up infections in a wide range of tissues. The bacteria have protein molecules sticking out from their surface that ward off the large white blood cells that roam the circulatory system looking for criminal insurgents and can develop an outer capsule that makes them even harder to attack. They are also equipped with the molecular equivalent of scissors, which snip at the parts of incoming defense cells that normally sniff out danger.

Avoiding being caught is great, but life as a disease-causing bug is even better if you can lock firmly onto target cells. Group A *streptococci* have a protein sticking that binds to cell walls. When this protein grabs a host cell, it triggers a process that causes the cell to draw it inside. An alternative option they use is to produce chemicals that break down the connections between cells, allowing the bacteria to spread rapidly through tissues.

Then comes the punch. Most strains of this bacterium produce one or more pyrogenic (heat-producing) toxins that induce fever. Some of these also cause the red rash that occurs with severe infections, and it is these toxins that can send a person's body into shock.

Symptoms and effects

Hopefully, an infection of these bacteria will just stay on the surface. A sore throat, for example, is most probably caused by *Str. pyogenes* living in the back of the mouth and releasing pyrogenic toxins. The immune system kills off the bacteria before they get any further—end of story. Alternatively, the bacteria can generate so much toxin that the person's body breaks out in a rash—they have scarlet fever, a disease that used to kill thousands of people a year. You can see the results of a skin infection with this bug when children get impetigo, a red and painful rash on their face.

Things turn distinctly nasty if the bacteria move deep into the tissues. In a situation called "necrotizing fasciitis," it can destroy fist-sized chunks of organs and flesh in days, leaving the person at best seriously ill. If the bacteria flood into the bloodstream, you land up with septic shock—another severely painful situation to be avoided if at all possible, which is accompanied by fever, vomiting, diarrhea, dizziness, confusion, and possible organ failure.

Developments in treatment

If you develop a major outbreak of this bug, your big hope is that doctors quickly find an antibiotic that is ideally suited to killing it. A rapid response is imperative and up to 10 days of specific antibiotics, maybe more, will be needed to clear it out.

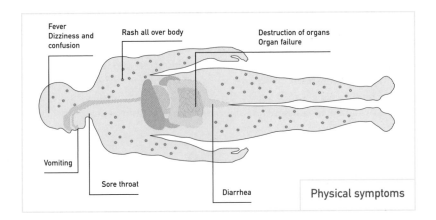

Physical symptoms

Clostridium Difficile

Agent: bacterium
Clostridium difficile
First recorded: 1977
Region: hospitals

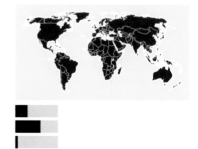

Infectivity	
Severity of illness	
Likelihood of dying if ill	
Bio-weapon threat	

You are unwell, so you take antibiotics, and a few days later you have diarrhea. There is a reasonable chance that the antibiotics have triggered a chain of events that have caused an explosion in the numbers of *Clostridium difficile* in your gut.

Origins

A healthy person's gut is packed with billions of bacteria. They are a necessary part of the process that breaks down food and makes the nutrients available to our bodies. These bacteria exist in a finely balanced ecosystem, and normally keep each others' populations in check, as well as fighting off harmful bacteria that may try to sneak in. This is all fine—until you take antibiotics. The chemical travels throughout the body, killing off bacteria wherever it goes. In the gut, the result is a change in the relative contribution made by different bugs. This appears to create an environment where *C. difficile* can thrive.

Given that loads of people in hospitals are taking antibiotics, it should be no surprise that hospitals are where many people develop *C. difficile*. However, there should be no grounds for complacency, as laboratory studies show that this particular bacteria has a great ability for jumping from patient to patient.

Symptoms and effects

The most common symptom is diarrhea, which is caused by toxins, given out by the bacteria, destroying parts of the gut's lining. The person also has gut pain and fever. In most people, the symptoms are not severe and they quickly recover, as long as they don't become dehydrated. Occasionally, people develop a more dangerous form of the disease in which the bowel becomes grossly dilated and may even tear—in the most extreme situations, this can be fatal.

Region of operation
Hospitals in developed countries are the best place to avoid if you want to give this bug the slip. Picking up this bacterium anywhere else is almost unheard of.

Historic outbreaks
In the first few years of the twenty-first century, the U.K. started a monitoring program to see how frequently these bacteria affected people in hospitals. Its recorded incidence therefore soared. Headline writers jumped to claim that we had a new outbreak of disease, but in reality we were just measuring an ongoing outbreak without any idea of whether health authorities were keeping it under control, winning the war, or letting things slip. It will take a decade of recording before we really know which of these is occurring.

Developments in treatment
The first step is to stop giving the antibiotic that enabled these bacteria to proliferate in the first place, then hit the *C. difficile* with one of the newer antibiotics, such as Vancomycin, that few bacteria have learned to resist. This should treat the problem that caused doctors to prescribe antibiotics in the

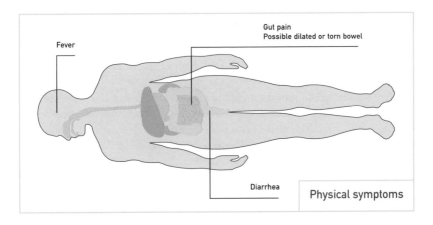

Fever

Gut pain
Possible dilated or torn bowel

Diarrhea

Physical symptoms

Helicobacter Pylori

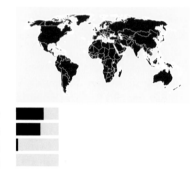

Agent: bacterium
Helicobacter pylori
First recorded: 1982
Region: global

Infectivity	████
Severity of illness	████
Likelihood of dying if ill	▌
Bio-weapon threat	

Once upon a time, doctors said that stress caused stomach ulcers. If you had a stomach ulcer, you needed to slow down, chill out, and take antacid tablets. Then two researchers discovered *Helicobacter pylori*.

Origins

In the 1980s, Australian medics and researchers Robin Warren and Barry Marshall had a hunch. They believed that stomach ulcers were not mainly due to stressed lifestyles, but to infection; more specifically, to infection with *H. pylori*. Warren was studying tissue samples taken from people's stomachs during clinical investigations. He spotted that half of the samples had a particular type of curved bacteria, and that these bacteria were always around when there was inflammation near by. His conclusion was that the bacteria were causing the inflammation. Marshall joined in Warren's research, and together they found a way of growing these curious bacteria in the laboratory. They then discovered that they could find them in almost all patients with gastric inflammation, duodenal ulcers, or gastric ulcers.

The medical community was slow to accept the idea that micro-organisms caused stomach ulcers, and the pharmaceutical community was very happy to continue selling antacid medications to sufferers. Frustrated, Warren came in to work one day in 1982 and swallowed a draft of *H. pylori*. Within days he was showing all the signs of having major stomach ulcers. He then swallowed a cocktail of antibiotics to clear them out, and the ulcers healed over. The world sat up and listened and two of the world's biggest selling drugs, the acid-suppressing Tagamet and Zantac, were no longer quite as valuable.

Symptoms and effects

A few days after a person has been infected, they have bouts of stomach pain, feel sick, and have flatulence and bad breath. These symptoms may last for a couple of years, but the infection can hang around for much longer.

It's not just ulcers that you need to worry about, though. *H. pylori* also leaves the stomach wall prone to developing cancer. There are also concerns that it could be one of the causes behind issues as varied as coronary heart disease, iron deficiency, anemia, and even sudden infant death syndrome.

Region of operation

As far as we know at the moment, humans are the only animals that harbor *H. pylori*, and quite how the bacteria manage to spread between people remains a mystery. Infection rates are higher among people who experienced poor and overcrowded living conditions when they were a child.

Developments in treatment

It's not always imperative to eradicate *H. pylori* if it is in your stomach, but if a doctor decides that you need to get rid of it then there are some successful steps that can be taken. Giving a one-week course of three different antibiotics wipes it out in 90 percent of people, and continued use of antibiotics can eventually clear it from most of the rest.

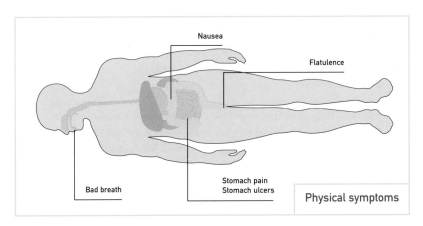

Nausea

Flatulence

Bad breath

Stomach pain
Stomach ulcers

Physical symptoms

Hepatitis C

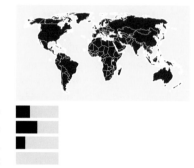

Agent: virus
Hepatits C virus (Family: *Flaviviridae*)
First recorded: 1989
Region: global

Infectivity	■
Severity of illness	■
Likelihood of dying if ill	■
Bio-weapon threat	

Hepatitis comes in various forms: A, B, C, D, and E. But don't be fooled by the similarity in the names. Although the viruses all attack the liver and so cause liver inflammation, or "hepatitis" in Latin, the five viruses are all very different. Hepatitis C is particularly nasty, and over the past 30 years it has emerged from being a shadowy enigma to becoming a worrying risk to health.

Origins

When hepatitis C was first identified, around 50,000 people were found in the U.S.A. alone with the virus on board. Knowing an enemy is the first step in eradicating it, and discovering that it could readily travel in donated blood gave health workers an insight into how to stop it. Since 1991, all donated blood has been screened for the virus, and contaminated blood is thrown out. As a result, infections have dropped to below 10,000 a year in the U.S.A.

Currently, an estimated 170 million people around the world have the disease. The main reason it hasn't been eradicated is that it piggybacks very successfully from one person to another if two or more people share a single hypodermic needle. About 20 percent of regular drug users become infected each year, so a long-term user is almost guaranteed to carry the virus.

This, coupled with the fact that some countries pay donors to give blood, gives rise to an interesting problem. Giving blood is a simple way of making money and drug users are always looking for a quick buck—but they are the very people you want to steer clear of when it comes to collecting blood that will eventually be handed on to someone who is already ill. It is one of the arguments for systems that stick to voluntary donation.

Symptoms and effects

It takes about eight weeks from the date of infection to the first time that a doctor would be able to carry out blood tests and detect that something is wrong with the liver. From that point, the person will probably start to feel weak, nauseous, and unwilling to eat. In half to three-quarters of infected people, the virus takes up permanent residence and is therefore referred to as a chronic or persistent infection. Over time, a range of physical damage starts to occur within the liver, including a breakdown of some of the ducts, inflammation of the lobes, and the development of abnormal blister-like follicles. As if that is not enough, the virus is also linked to liver cancer.

Historic outbreaks

Egypt has a particular problem with hepatitis C, with infection rates as high as 30 percent. This is due to a 1960s vaccination campaign against bilharzia, which used re-usable needles without sterilizing them between patients.

Developments in treatment

Alpha-interferon is the only real hope. Given three times a week for six to 12 months, it can remove the virus from the body. It is then up to the body to try to rebuild its liver. This is only possible if the damage is minor—if it is more severe, the person has to wait for a liver transplant.

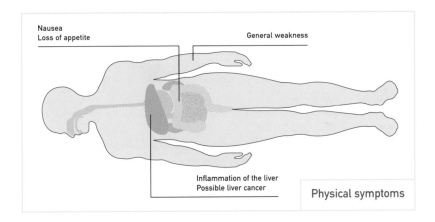

Nausea
Loss of appetite

General weakness

Inflammation of the liver
Possible liver cancer

Physical symptoms

Rotavirus

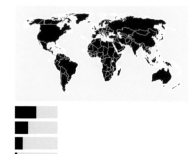

Agent: virus
Group A rotavirus
First recorded: 1980s in China
Region: global

Infectivity	
Severity of illness	
Likelihood of dying if il	
Bio-weapon threat	

Rotavirus accounts for more cases of infant diarrhea than any other disease. Most of the children who suffer from it are aged between three months and two years. The scale of the problem can be seen in the fact that an estimated 600,000 children a year die of it, and three million children in the U.S. develop diarrhea after becoming infected, with 55,000 of these needing hospital care to help them survive it.

Origins

Rotaviruses get their name because of their appearance. Viewed through an electron microscope, they are wheel-like, and *rota* is Latin for wheel. They are wrapped up in two coats of protein, which enables them to survive well even outside a human host. The virus leaves the body through feces, and poor hygiene enables it to move rapidly to other friends and family.

Washing your hands after using the toilet or helping a child use the toilet is a basic first step of prevention, but the virus is robust and will withstand the assault of most soaps and cleansers. Washing your hands will therefore reduce the number of viruses left behind, but not eliminate them.

Symptoms and effects

The gut is lined with cells that have microscopic finger-like projections sticking out of them. These massively increase the intestine's surface area and enable it to absorb nutrients as they flow by. Once in the gut, rotaviruses move into the cells at the tips of these projections and use the machinery inside them to build new copies of themselves. Between 10 and 12 hours after infecting the cells the viruses break out, destroying the tips. This leaves the gut unable to absorb material, so it flows straight through, appearing as diarrhea.

Over a few days, your immune system cuts in and destroys the viruses, ridding you of the disease and protecting you from this particular virus in the future. Sadly, there are many different sub-types of rotavirus, so you can easily be infected by the next variant that does the rounds.

Region of operation

The virus exists all around the world, but causes most problems where people do not have clean water. To survive the disease, all you need to do is keep alive for a few days, but with fluids pouring out and the gut much less capable of absorbing water, the struggle is to keep hydrated. If you are in a hot country, the need is even more extreme. 1.4 ounces (40 g) and 0.1 ounce (3.5 g) salt in 2.1 pints (1 liter) of clean water is all that is needed to keep most children alive. Sadly, even that is not available in many places.

Developments in treatment

Researchers have had difficulty coming up with a vaccine that protects people from all of the different forms of rotavirus. In 1998, a vaccine was released, but it was soon withdrawn because it seemed to damage gut development. Rehydration remains the only option.

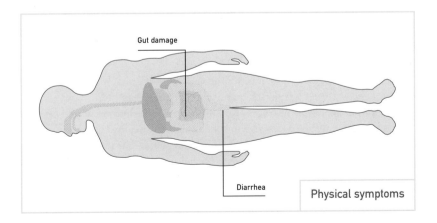

Gut damage

Diarrhea

Physical symptoms

SARS (Severe Acute Respiratory Syndrome)

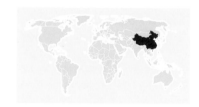

Agent: virus
SARS-associated coronavirus
(SARS-CoV) (Family: *Viverridae*)
First recorded: November 2002
Region: mainly China

Infectivity	
Severity of illness	
Likelihood of dying if ill	
Bio-weapon threat	

It doesn't happen often, but every now and again a new disease appears as if from nowhere. The problems are immense if it turns out to spread easily from person to person. Paradoxically, it is easier to track down a disease if it makes people seriously ill within days or hours of becoming infected—at least that way investigators can follow its spread and isolate people who appear to be carrying the agent.

In the case of SARS, authorities had to scramble fast to break the chain of infection, while at the same time trying to make sense of the nature of the newly emerged disease.

Origins

On November 16, 2002 a man in his 40s went into hospital in Foshan, China. It seemed as if he had pneumonia. He recovered and went home—an utterly unremarkable event, except that other people in the area started getting ill. The Chinese authorities were either unaware that they had a novel disease on their hands, or were keen to cover it up in the hope that it would go away as quickly and quietly as it had arrived. The net result was that, in doing nothing to combat the disease, they let it spread.

That spread came to the world's attention when, on February 21, 2003, 64-year-old professor of nephrology at Zhongsham University Liu Jianlun checked into room 911 at the Metropole Hotel in Hong Kong. He'd spent the previous weeks treating people with a mystery illness, and had then traveled to Hong Kong for a family wedding. Almost as soon as he arrived, he realized he had the symptoms of the disease and took himself to the local hospital. He died 11 days later. The doctor had suffered his patient's fate.

Not only that, but he had also left a trail of viruses behind him. Hotel visitors who had shared the elevator with Liu took the bug to Hanoi, Bangkok, Toronto, and Singapore. By April 1, 2003, Hong Kong had 685 reported cases and 16 deaths, and the epidemic was escalating. A global scientific effort

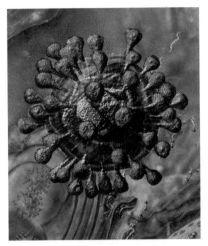

Above Artwork of a SARS virus particle inside a cell. Like all viruses, it cannot replicate by itself; instead, it infects a cell and uses that cell's machinery to produce more copies of the virus.

played catch-up, and in April discovered that the infection was being caused by a form of coronavirus—an irregularly shaped and poorly understood viral particle.

There was a palpable sense of fear as infra-red scanners in airports and railway stations tried to detect anyone with a fever and stop them traveling. The World Health Organization issued a global alert on March 12, 2003, followed by a health alert by the United States Centers for Disease Control and Prevention. Residents of entire tower blocks and districts were placed in quarantine, and international conferences were cancelled. However, with knowledge of the foe, authorities could start to contain it. By the time that infections came to an end in July, the illness had been spread by international travelers to more than two dozen countries in Asia, North America, South America, and Europe. The total number of people affected around the world had risen to 8,098 ill and 774 dead, of which eight cases showed up in the U.S.A. And then SARS seemed to disappear.

Symptoms and effects

Symptoms usually appeared two to ten days following exposure. On the face of it, people with SARS just had a nasty form of flu—symptoms included fever, lethargy, cough, sore throat, and muscular aches and pains—with the added inconvenience that some also developed diarrhea. The only symptom common to all patients was a temperature above 100.4°F (38°C). However, it was only after their death that the true destructive nature of the beast became clear. All sufferers had massively reduced numbers of the white cells that normally fight infections, as well as depleted reserves of platelets, which help the blood to clot when tissues are damaged. Add these two together, and the victim is left in a highly vulnerable state.

Postmortem surveys found that victims' lungs had started to collapse and leak fluid into the airspaces. They found large areas of dead tissue inside the lymph glands and the spleen, as well as blood cells leaking into the tissues of the heart, kidneys, lungs, liver, adrenal glands, and some areas of the brain. While many viruses target only a few organs, this one operates with biological "shock and awe."

Region of operation

Like many viral diseases, the SARS virus appears to have existed in wild mammals such as the masked palm civet and Chinese ferret badgers, animals that are sold for food in some exotic meat markets in Eastern countries. These animals provide a safe haven for the virus without themselves becoming ill, and SARS only appeared after a small change in its genes occurred that allowed it to venture into humans and spread from person to person.

Once out and about, the SARS virus can potentially operate anywhere in the world. However, it needs to be in a fairly densely populated area in order to spread well. If you are infected and cough into your hand, the fine spray of saliva that mists your palm will be loaded with viruses. Touch a surface like a door handle, and the viruses will be transferred. Other people grabbing the handle will pick them up, and, if they inadvertently rub their eyes, pick their noses, or put their fingers in their mouth, the virus can come on board.

The features that limit this means of transmission are temperature, humidity, and sunlight. In dark, damp, and warm conditions, the virus can survive for hours. On a hot, dry surface in full sunlight, it lasts for minutes.

Development of treatment

The bad news is that, as with all viruses, the only effective treatment is to support the person in the hope that they recover. SARS was typically treated with fever-reducing drugs, extra oxygen and ventilatory support where needed. The good news is that this is not an issue, because at the moment the virus has stopped attacking us. The last known case was reported in China on May 2, 2004, and the epidemic strain that caused so many deaths worldwide in 2003 has not been seen outside of the laboratory since then. The W.H.O. declared the disease "eradicated" in May 2005, making it only the second disease in the history of mankind to receive this label (the other being smallpox).

Potential threat to civilization

There is very little chance of SARS being used as a terror weapon, because it is so difficult to track down. No one knows where it came from, so it would be virtually impossible for any terror organization to culture it from some native source, and even if you did get hold of a sample it is technically very difficult to culture.

That said, the last people who were infected with it were scientists who were working on it in a laboratory at the National University of Singapore. While stocks of it exist, there is always the possibility of an accidental release. Or, presumably, it could always just re-appear from the wild.

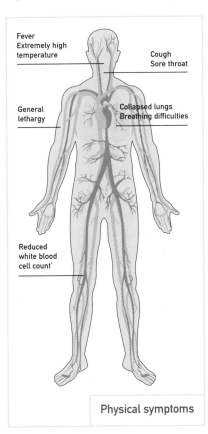

Fever
Extremely high temperature

Cough
Sore throat

General lethargy

Collapsed lungs
Breathing difficulties

Reduced white blood cell count

Physical symptoms

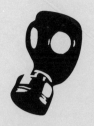

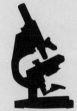

Part Two:
Airborne Diseases

Whooping Cough

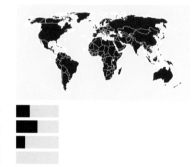

Agent: bacterium
Bordetella sp.
First recorded: 2.5 million years ago
Region: global

Infectivity	
Severity of illness	
Likelihood of dying if ill	
Bio-weapon threat	

Three different but closely related species of bacteria cause whooping cough: *Bordetella pertusis*, *B. parapertusis* and *B. bronchiseptica*. Between them they kill over 300,000 people a year.

Origins

Recent studies have given some fascinating insights into these species. By looking at the number of genetic mutations in different bacteria that belong to a single species, scientists are able to estimate the amount of time for which a species has been around. In this case, there is every indication that they first attacked hominids around 2.5 million years ago. They have therefore had plenty of time to perfect their menace.

Symptoms and effects

Typically, a child has many bouts of severe coughing each day, with symptom-free periods in between. During the paroxysms of coughing, the child's tongue is pushed far forwards, and fluids stream from his or her eyes and nose. Just as the face turns blue, the child manages to cough up a lump of phlegm and, with a clear throat, draws in a massive draft of air, creating a high-pitched "whooping" sound.

The bacteria bind themselves to the outer layer of cells in the lungs and release a toxin that paralyzes the microscopic hair-like brushes that normally sweep the lungs clean. With these immobilized, the bacteria are less likely to be thrown out, but there is also no way of clearing the mucus that the lungs constantly produce. This collects until it starts to block the airways and needs to be coughed away. If the patient can't clear the mucus, the lung collapses. The only route now is a few days in intensive care, as without that support death is not far away.

Historic outbreaks

Epidemics of the disease tend to occur every four to five years. Once an outbreak has started, it is difficult to contain unless a large proportion of the population is vaccinated. Antibiotics are only partially effective because the bacteria never enter the body but instead sit on the outside of the lung's lining, so many will not meet the antibiotics even if the patient takes some. On top of this, each cough sends thousands of bacteria-laden droplets into the air. Sharing a house with an infected sibling gives you a 90 percent chance of infection, while going to school with an infected classmate carries a 50 percent chance.

Developments in treatment

There is a vaccine, but it will only stamp out the disease if it has near total uptake within a community. Pre-unification Germany provides an intriguing test case. In the former West Germany, vaccination was voluntary and uptake was low, but in the former East Germany it was compulsory and in 1989 coverage was 95 percent. Between 1980 and 1990, the incidence of whooping cough was 100 times higher in the West compared to the East.

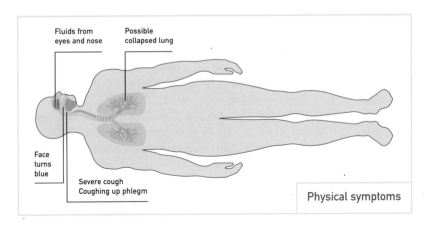

Fluids from eyes and nose

Possible collapsed lung

Face turns blue

Severe cough
Coughing up phlegm

Physical symptoms

Common Cold

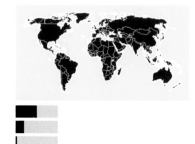

Agent: virus (Family: *picornavirus*)
Rhinoviruses
First recorded: antiquity
Region: global

Infectivity		
Severity of illness		
Likelihood of dying if ill		
Bio-weapon threat		

Approximately 95 percent of normal adults become infected when researchers drop viruses into their noses. It might not always seem this way, because out of the people who become infected, only 75 percent develop cold symptoms. The other 25 percent have the virus growing in their nose, but have no symptoms.

Why some people do not develop cold symptoms is a mystery, but it may be that these are the people with unusually poor abilities to produce the messages within cells that are needed to trigger symptoms. If this theory is correct, people with active immune systems may be more prone to developing cold symptoms than people with less active immune systems.

Origins
There are over 100 different cold viruses, but as a group, *rhinoviruses* are the most important because they cause at least half of all colds. The name comes from the Greek word *rhino*, which means nose.

Symptoms and effects
The symptoms of a common cold include a feeling that your nose is blocked, but at the same time you need to sneeze, and your nose constantly runs with watery mucus. You have a sore or scratchy throat, a cough, a hoarse voice, mild headaches, feverishness, and chilliness. In general, you don't feel well. Adults average two to three colds per year and children six to ten, depending on their age and exposure. Children's noses are the major source of cold viruses. On average, the symptoms last for around a week, though a bad bout can go on for a couple of weeks.

Region of operation

The common cold is one of the virus world's success stories. It travels everywhere, and because immunity from each attack only lasts for around four years, there is always a population of people ready and waiting to give it a home in their noses. In the U.S.A., which has a population of just under 300 million, around 22 million school days are lost each year due to the common cold.

Developments in treatment

Nobel Prize winner Linus Pauling was convinced that vitamin C could ward off the common cold. A huge industry now works on that claim, but several large-scale research studies have started to question it. They have tested the theory by dividing people into two groups. One group is given vitamin C tablets, while the other is given a placebo (a tablet that looks and tastes the same, but contains none of the active ingredient—in this case, vitamin C). Both groups had similar numbers of colds and cold symptoms.

Potential threat to civilization

Isolated communities of hunter-gatherers, indigenous rain forest dwellers, and Australian Aboriginals have all suffered greatly when a Western traveler has arrived and introduced the common cold. In some cases, the outbreak of disease was so severe that entire communities were destroyed.

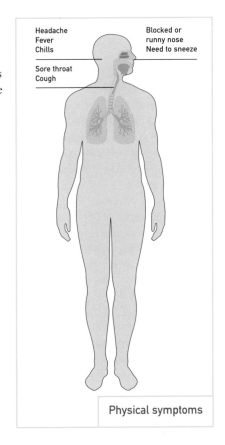

Headache
Fever
Chills

Blocked or
runny nose
Need to sneeze

Sore throat
Cough

Physical symptoms

English Sweating Sickness

Agent: unknown
First recorded: 1486
Region: England

Infectivity	■■□□
Severity of illness	■■□□
Likelihood of dying if ill	■■□□
Bio-weapon threat	□□□□

In the summer of 1485, Henry Tudor had just landed at Milford Haven, England, about to win the Battle of Bosworth Field and become King Henry VII of England. However, war was not the only way of dying quickly in England that summer, because a new sickness had appeared. It wasn't the plague—the symptoms were wrong and it killed too quickly—and, despite various attempts by historians, no one has quite decided what it was. At the time, the locals called it "Sudor Anglais," or "English Sweat," but the symptoms led to it being renamed "English Sweating Sickness."

Symptoms and effects

The sixteenth-century English medics John Caius and Thomas Forestier described what happened to the people who caught this disease. There were six separate "signes or tokens:" headache and muscle pain, vomiting, delirium, heart palpitations, paralysis, and breathlessness, and then death. In contrast to plague, victims had no "buboes" or other skin signs. The disease moved rapidly, with victims going from first symptom to death within 12 to 24 hours.

Region of operation

This disease was pretty much only recorded in England, although there were some reports of a similar condition breaking out sporadically in northern France. It is now unknown anywhere in the world.

The disease operated mainly in rural areas, although at times outbreaks were recorded in cities like London, Oxford, and Cambridge. Strangely, the records show that within local communities or families you could see batches of men dying, or batches of women, but seldom a balance of both sexes. Because of the way that people lived at the time, this strongly suggests that the disease was moving person to person as an airborne infection, and because of the pace of its attack and the nature of the symptoms, it was probably viral in nature.

This sweating sickness also moved from settlement to settlement along lines of communication and trade, in a pattern similar to that seen for diseases spread by rodent-borne insects like fleas.

Historic outbreaks

By searching through church records of burials from the fifteenth and sixteenth centuries, historians have discovered that there were five distinct outbreaks of this sweating sickness: 1485, 1508, 1517, 1528, and 1551.

Potential threat to civilization

The speed of the disease brings both bad and good news. The downside is that if you get it, tragedy is not far away, but the benefit of this is that the disease doesn't have much time to spread to others. Consequently, outbreaks of these rapidly developing infections tend to be self-limiting. This lessens their threat, but does not diminish their terror.

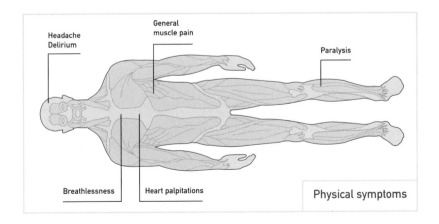

Headache
Delirium

General
muscle pain

Paralysis

Breathlessness

Heart palpitations

Physical symptoms

Measles

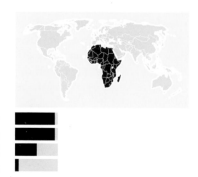

Agent: virus
Morbillivirus
First recorded: ancient
Region: predominantly Africa

Infectivity	
Severity of illness	
Likelihood of dying if ill	
Bio-weapon threat	

This severe and highly contagious condition could be on the endangered list, so long as each generation of parents vaccinates their children. The vaccine became available in the early 1960s, and rates of infection and death plummeted. While there is still a long way to go, we are heading in the right direction. In 1999, for example, an estimated 871,000 people were killed by the disease, but by 2004 this had dropped to 454,000, with half of those deaths occuring in Africa.

Origins

There are reports of diseases that sound similar to measles dating back to at least 600 B.C.E., but the first scientific description of the disease and its distinction from smallpox came when Persian physician Ibn Razi (860–932 C.E.) published a book entitled *Smallpox and Measles*. The virus that causes measles, *morbillivirus*, was isolated in 1954 and the first vaccines became available in 1963.

Symptoms and effects

Measles is spread through fluids from an infected person's nose and mouth, either directly or through droplets in the air. It is a highly contagious disease—around 90 percent of people who have no immunity to measles and who are sharing a house with an infected person will catch it.

Some nine to eleven days after becoming infected, the person starts feeling tired and exhausted. He or she develops a high fever, runny eyes, and swollen eyelids. Soon the person starts to dislike light, and begins to have cold-like symptoms. After three or four days, a bright red rash breaks out on the forehead and face. It then travels down the neck and trunk, reaching the feet within three days. This rash, which can be itchy, changes color from dark brown to red over the course of the infection. After three days it will start to go away. The infected person will remain contagious from the appearance of the first symptoms until three to five days after the rash disappears.

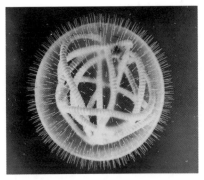

Above The measles virus consists of an outer envelope studded with small, spiky projections, a coiled-rope formation capsid (protein shell), and the nucleic acids—which carry the genetic code of the virus—wound in a spiral inside.

If the symptoms stop here, then all is well. The problems start if other symptoms appear. Many victims will get diarrhea and ear infections, and quite a few develop pneumonia and bronchitis. One in 200 suffer from convulsions and fits, and one in 1000 meningitis. These complications lead to one in 2,500 children dying from the disease, with one in 8,000 surviving but with severe brain damage.

Region of operation

In developed countries, most children are vaccinated when they are 18 months old, usually as part of a three-part M.M.R. vaccine (measles, mumps and rubella). As a result, the disease is relatively rare in these areas and the fatality rate is very low. However, measles is still very much a part of life and death in developing countries where vaccination is limited, and people living in countries of Africa that have poor infrastructures have been particularly hard to reach. This lack of immunization, combined with malnutrition, means that fatality rates can be as high as 10 percent.

Historic outbreaks

A single piece of research published in a U.K. medical journal in 1998 suggested that there may be a link between the vaccine used to prevent measles and some stomach conditions. Many other studies failed to confirm this link, but the fears of this remote risk led to many parents refusing the vaccine—despite the fact that doing so put their children at much greater risk of catching a life-threatening disease. With vaccination rates dropping, there is now a high risk of an epidemic, and the possibility of this was highlighted in the U.K. in early 2006 when a child suddenly died of measles. This made headlines because it was the first measles-related death in the U.K. for 10 years.

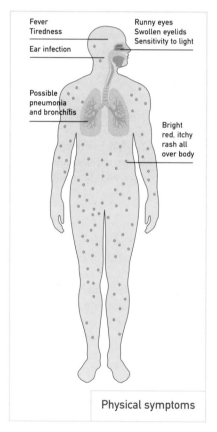

Fever
Tiredness
Ear infection
Possible pneumonia and bronchitis

Runny eyes
Swollen eyelids
Sensitivity to light
Bright red, itchy rash all over body

Physical symptoms

Developments in treatment

There is no specific treatment for measles—rest and support are generally enough to promote recovery. Vaccination is therefore the only way to try to protect yourself, and requires just two doses of an inexpensive, safe, and widely available vaccine. This, however, does not guarantee that the vaccinated child cannot get measles; it only makes around 90 percent of them immune to the disease. To make vaccination strategies work, you need the entire population to take the vaccine. That way, while there are a few people who will not have become immune, they will be spread so thinly throughout the population that the virus can't jump from one to another. Without the ability to travel, the virus will die out. Deciding not to go along with a vaccination program not only puts your child at risk, but also increases the risk for everyone else.

Tuberculosis (TB)

Agent: bacterium
Mycobacterium tuberculosis complex
First recorded: antiquity
Region: global

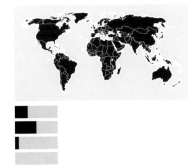

Infectivity	
Severity of illness	
Likelihood of dying if ill	
Bio-weapon threat	

Tuberculosis is one of the most deadly and most common infectious diseases operating in the world today. According to World Health Organization estimates, one-third of the world's population has been infected with tuberculosis bacteria, and about 100 million people catch the disease for the first time each year. Of these, around 8 to 10 million develop signs of the disease and 3 million die.

Although most cases are found in the developing world, a growing number of people in developed countries are contracting the disease because they have weakened immune systems—typically due to taking immunosuppressant drugs or because of HIV/AIDS.

Origins

Tuberculosis has been present in human society since antiquity. Skeletal remains from around 4000 B.C.E. show marks that are characteristic of TB, and the spines of Egyptian mummies from 3000–2400 B.C.E. also show signs that the bacteria had infected the body. Writings found in India indicate that the disease was there in 2000 B.C.E., and archeological evidence suggests that it was also in the Americas at a similar time.

The specific species of bacteria that caused the disease was eventually tracked down by German physician Robert Koch, who received the 1905 Nobel Prize in Physiology and Medicine for his troubles. He, however, thought that bovine (cattle) and human tuberculosis were quite separate diseases. Once doctors discovered that they were related, the dairy industry started heating, or "pasteurizing," milk before selling it. This removed one of

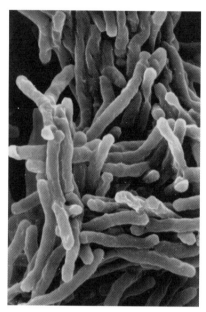

Above The *mycobacterium tuberculosis* bacteria, the main cause of TB in humans.

the key routes by which humans became infected.

Symptoms and effects

Tuberculosis used to be known as consumption or wasting disease, as it seemed to consume the body from within. The disease most commonly affects the lungs, with the symptoms including cough, chest pain, fever, night sweats, appetite loss, weight loss, and fatigue. This species of bacteria has a number of properties that make it difficult to attack. To start with, many people don't show any symptoms for years or decades after the initial infection—the bacteria just sit in the lung and wait. Quite what triggers their activation varies from person to person, but it often occurs when someone is knocked down by a different illness.

At this point, colonies start growing inside the lung, creating zones of dead and damaged tissue, and materials released from the bacteria trigger fevers and muscle wastage. As the regions of damage expand, they eventually break into the airpipes, and the bacteria flood into the mucus. Therefore, each time the person coughs, millions of bacteria are launched into the air. These patients are referred to as being "open" or "infective," and they spread the disease through the droplets they expel into the air when they cough, sneeze, spit, or speak.

Once the infection can break out of the lungs, it can also travel within a person, setting up colonies in the mouth and larynx. Swallowed bacteria cause problems in the gut, and others move to the bladder and kidney, as well as establishing themselves in the skin of the face and neck. If untreated, these can lead to permanent scars.

Region of operation

Tuberculosis thrives where people are packed together in poor living conditions. Prisons in developing countries are particular hot-spots as people are poorly fed, often unwell, and living in close proximity to one another. Ventilation is often poor so one inmate breathes in the bacteria-filled droplets that another coughs out.

Tuberculosis also attacks people with weakened immune systems, such as those suffering from HIV/AIDS or anyone taking immunosuppressant drugs. This, combined with the neglect of TB control programs and increased migration, has led to a resurgence of the disease, and the W.H.O. declared TB a global health emergency in 1993.

Developments in treatment

In 1906, French scientists Albert Calmette and Camille Guerin developed the Bacillus of Calmette and Guerinin, or BCG, vaccine. This was first used on humans in 1921. While this introduced a method of helping to prevent people from catching the disease, it wasn't until 1946 that the antibiotic streptomycin arrived, and gave the hope of killing bacteria that had set up an infection.

Over the years, the bacteria have developed resistance to many antibiotics. Ridding a person of tuberculosis now means giving them a combination of antibiotics for up to six months.

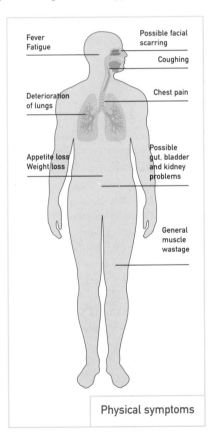

Fever
Fatigue

Possible facial scarring

Coughing

Deterioration of lungs

Chest pain

Appetite loss
Weight loss

Possible gut, bladder and kidney problems

General muscle wastage

Physical symptoms

Legionnaires' Disease

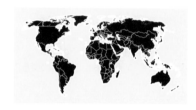

Agent: bacterium
Legionella pneumophila
First recorded: 1976
Region: inside air-conditioned buildings

Infectivity	
Severity of illness	
Likelihood of dying if ill	
Bio-weapon threat	

The built environment brings many advantages, but the more technology you cram inside, the more there is to go wrong. Interestingly, heating, humidifying, and air-conditioning systems provide a perfect home for *Legionella pneumophila*, a bug that can infect and attack the lungs.

Origins

This disease was first discovered in 1976 among a group of elderly men attending an American Legion Convention in Philadelphia, Pennsylvania. This outbreak caused an element of panic as no one knew why so many men at one convention were coming down with breathing difficulties. It took a year to track down the bug, and the culprit was found to be a rod-shaped bacterium. The only known way of picking up this bug is to inhale an aerosol of fine water droplets that are laced with the bacteria.

Symptoms and effects

After an incubation period of between two and 10 days, *L. pneumophila* starts to trigger a fever and make it hard to breathe as the airspaces in the lungs fill with mucus. The fever rises until the victims start to become confused and hallucinate; they may even have fits. The fatality rate can be as high as 80 percent in people who are not treated and have poor immune systems, but in healthy people who receive good medical care it can be reduced to between five and ten percent.

Region of operation

These bacteria need to get into water droplets before moving into humans. This means that hot tubs and Jacuzzis are high-risk places if you want to be sure of avoiding the disease. Heating and air-conditioning systems are often lined with condensation and, if they are not cleaned frequently, can introduce disease.

Historic outbreaks

There have been plenty of small-scale outbreaks since 1976. In August 2002, an outbreak of Legionnaires' disease linked to a council-run sports center in the town of Barrow-in-Furness, Cumbria, U.K., led to seven deaths and 170 people falling ill. In September 2005, 21 elderly people died as a result of a Legionnaires' outbreak associated with a nursing home in Toronto, Canada.

Each outbreak seems to bring as many lawyers running to the scene as health-care professionals, the general view being that good maintenance should be able to keep this bug away.

Developments in treatment

This needs to be taken seriously, and most treatment involves injecting high doses of antibiotics into the bloodstream. Erythromycin is the most commonly used antibiotic for this disease, although taking the more recently developed azithromycin as tablets or in a syrup could become the treatment of choice.

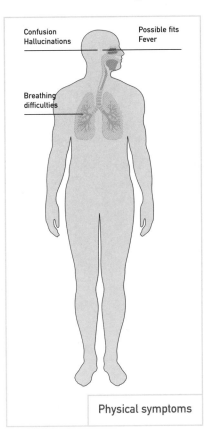

Confusion
Hallucinations

Possible fits
Fever

Breathing difficulties

Physical symptoms

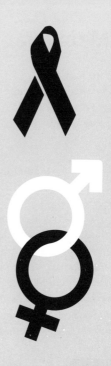

Part Three:

Sexually Transmitted Diseases

Chlamydia

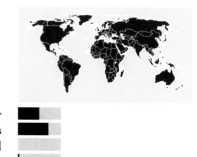

Agent: bacterium
Chlamydia trachomatis
First recorded: 1960s
Region: global

Infectivity	■■■
Severity of illnes	■■■
Likelihood of dying if ill	■■
Bio-weapon threat	▎

Chlamydia is an increasingly common sexually transmitted disease (STD). It can be transmitted during vaginal, anal, or oral sex. Chlamydia can also be passed from an infected mother to her baby during childbirth.

Any sexually active person can be infected with chlamydia bacteria, and the greater the number of sexual partners a person has, the greater his or her risk of infection. Teenage girls are particularly vulnerable because their cervix (opening to the uterus) is not fully matured. Since chlamydia can be transmitted by oral or anal sex, men who have same-sex intercourse are also at risk.

Symptoms and effects

Caused by the bacterium *Chlamydia trachomatis*, this illness can damage a woman's reproductive organs even though she may show no symptoms of an infection. The damage can be irreversible and can lead to the woman being infertile for the rest of her life.

In women who do experience symptoms, they usually appear one to three weeks after exposure. If the bacteria enter via the vagina, they initially infect the cervix and the urethra (the tube that brings urine from the kidneys.) It is possible for these women to have an abnormal vaginal discharge, or a burning sensation when urinating. When the infection spreads from the cervix, it damages the fallopian tubes, which carry sperm to meet eggs, and then let early embryos travel down into the uterus. This may lead to pain low in the back, nausea, fever, pain during intercourse, or bleeding between menstrual periods.

The first that many women know about this infection is many years later, either when they cannot get pregnant, or when an embryo forms but establishes itself inside the abdominal cavity instead of in the womb. This occurs because, whether or not a woman experiences symptoms, the bacteria in the fallopian tubes damage the cells making up this delicate part of the reproductive system. If the tubes are completely blocked, no sperm can pass up to meet the egg, so no fertilization occurs. If they are only partially blocked, sperm can travel up to fertilize the egg, but the fertilized egg cannot move down into the womb. In this case, the embryo will develop in the body cavity, and this "ectopic" pregnancy will almost certainly kill the woman if it is not removed.

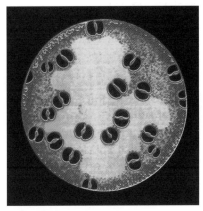

Above The kidney-shaped chlamydia bacterium is typically found in pairs.

Alternatively, these bacteria can set up an infection in the rectum, either by traveling there from a woman's vagina, or by being introduced during anal sex in men or women. This can cause rectal pain, discharge, or bleeding.

Men normally have no symptoms, but those that do release discharge from their penises or have burning sensations when urinating. Some also have burning and itching around the opening of the penis. A few men develop pain and swelling in the testicles. Chlamydia can also be found in the throats of women and men having oral sex with an infected partner.

Because chlamydia can infect babies as they are being born, it is one of the leading causes of early infant pneumonia and eye infections.

Region of operation
Any society in which men and women are sexually active with multiple partners is at risk. Estimates suggest that 2.8 million Americans are infected with chlamydia each year, and somewhere around 100,000 women a year in the U.S.A. become infertile as a result of these infections. In the U.K., just over 100,000 women and men were found to be infected in 2004, and health experts believe that this is just the tip of the iceberg, as many more will have

picked up the bacteria without knowing it. As with all sexually transmitted diseases, sex workers throughout the world are at particular risk of having and spreading the infection. A recent World Health Organization survey discovered that almost 60 percent of women sex workers in China were infected with the bacterium, as were 10 percent of truck drivers. Similar surveys of sex workers in the towns of Port Moresby and Lae in the Philippines found that 30 percent of women carried chlamydia.

Developments in treatment

The good news is that the bacteria are easily killed by antibiotics—but you need to know that they are there to ask for treatment. The only way to know this is to analyze samples of urine or take swabs from suspected sites of infection. If an infection is found in one person, it is important to trace all other recent sexual partners so that they can receive treatment as well.

Potential threat to civilization

It is difficult to know whether rates of infection are soaring, or whether recently introduced monitoring is picking up an epidemic that has been with us for decades. Either way, a disease that is silently making many young women infertile is not good news for any civilization.

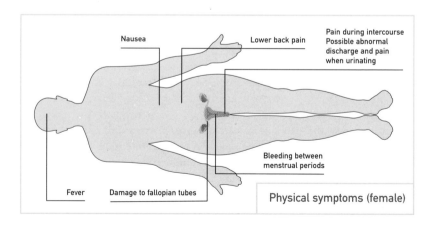

Nausea

Lower back pain

Pain during intercourse
Possible abnormal
discharge and pain
when urinating

Bleeding between
menstrual periods

Fever

Damage to fallopian tubes

Physical symptoms (female)

HIV/AIDS

Agent: virus (Family: *Retroviridae*)
Human immunodeficiency virus
First recorded: 1959
Region: global

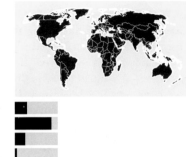

Infectivity	
Severity of illness	
Likelihood of dying if ill	
Bio-weapon threat	

One of the most contentious diseases currently roaming the globe is the breakdown of a person's immune system caused by the human immuno-deficiency virus (HIV). This virally triggered, acquired immunodeficiency syndrome (AIDS) has killed more than 25 million people since 1981, and has orphaned at least 12 million children in Africa alone.

Origins

HIV/AIDS came to the world's attention in 1981 when unusually high numbers of gay men in America started to develop rare cancers and did not respond to treatment for normally curable diseases. At first, health advisors said that this disease was completely confined to male homosexual communities, but by December that year it was clear that drug users were also at risk.

During the following year, some health professionals started calling the syndrome "gay compromise syndrome" or "gay-related immune deficiency," and by July 1982, over 450 cases had been reported in 23 states. By the end of the summer, reports of the disease infecting heterosexual men and women, as well as those who had hemophilia, meant that a new name was needed that removed any notion that it was confined to people of any particular sexual orientation, or that it could be transmitted solely by unprotected sex. AIDS became the name that stuck.

Over the last few decades, scientists have argued over how this scourge came into existence. One of the things that is clear is that its history goes back further than 1981. Trawling through archived blood samples has revealed that a man living in what is now the Democratic Republic of Congo had the virus

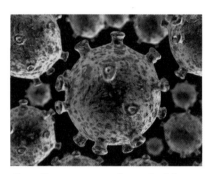

Above Computer-generated artwork of the HIV virus.

in his body back in 1959, and it was also found in samples from an American teenager who died in St. Louis in 1969. Where the virus came from has been the subject of best-selling books, court cases and huge international seminars—but there is still no firm conclusion. The most widely accepted theory is that it is a virus that has existed in simian monkeys in West Africa, and which jumped to humans after hunters ate infected meat. Strong evidence exists showing that humans who eat bush meat are at risk of picking up exotic viruses, which makes many people call for a complete ban on this element of the meat market.

Once it was in the population, the virus may have been spread from person to person by mass vaccination programs that occurred in the 1950s, which did not use disposable needles. Once the needle had been inserted into a person with the virus, there was a good chance that the virus would be passed to many of those who stood behind them in the queue. Before the source of the disease was tracked down, people with diseases like hemophilia, which are treated by giving repeated blood transfusions, were at particular risk. When a person with HIV gave a blood donation, they were also handing over the virus.

Undoubtedly, HIV's ability to be transmitted during sexual intercourse, coupled with a rise in the number of sexual partners with whom people interact, has been a cause for the explosive spread of the disease. This is exacerbated in male homosexual communities, as the virus seems to find it very easy to gain entry through anal sexual intercourse. Another reason why the HIV virus has been so successful at spreading is that it can infect a person for years before it causes symptoms, but during this period it can be passed to others.

Symptoms and effects

The most dangerous thing about HIV is that it attacks the immune system, the body's defense system that protects it from disease. With the defense system at reduced capacity, the body has less chance of getting rid of HIV, and it also lays the person open to attack from other diseases. One result of this is the escalating number of people suffering from tuberculosis, many of whom have succumbed to the disease because they were previously infected with HIV.

Developments in treatment

Antiviral therapy is beginning to come on to the market, but none of the products is completely effective. One of the problems is that, as viruses duplicate themselves, they introduce minor changes into the genetic code of the new generation. This constant mutation will produce individual viruses that can beat the antiviral drug and survive. If nothing is done, such drug-resistant strains will come to dominate the viral population.

In the most powerful treatment regime, termed "highly active antiretroviral therapy" (HAART), people take a combination of three or more different antiviral drugs. The idea is that, while a virus may mutate to evade one drug, the chances of it learning how to simultaneously tackle all three is very slight. Such mutants will still be eradicated.

While the aim of antiviral therapy is to rid a person of the virus, the best that normally happens is that the treatment slows down the progress of the disease. So, don't count on science to keep you safe from this one.

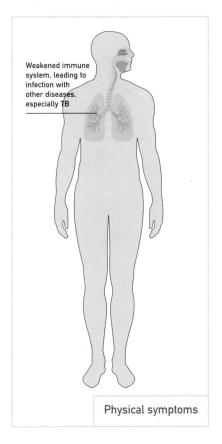

Weakened immune system, leading to infection with other diseases, especially TB

Physical symptoms

Herpes

Agent: Virus (Family: *Herpesviridae*)
Herpes simplex virus
First recorded: antiquity
Region: global

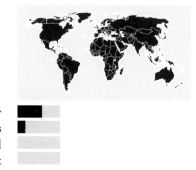

Infectivity	
Severity of illness	
Likelihood of dying if ill	
Bio-weapon threat	

The ancient Greek philosopher Hippocrates was one of the first people to describe a skin disease that sounds like herpes simplex, and it appears that the disease is named after the Greek word *herpes*, which means "to creep or crawl," in reference to the spreading nature of the herpetic skin lesions. However, it was only in 1893 that Parisian doctor Jean Baptiste Emile Vidal recognized that the disease was transmitted by a virus from one person to another. We now know that the same viruses are responsible for conditions like cold sores and genital herpes.

Symptoms and effects

There are two different versions of herpes simplex virus, HSV-1 and HSV-2, and HSV-2 is the one that most frequently infects the genital regions. These viruses set up an initial infection that creates a "vesicle," which is an inflating breakdown of skin cells. The cells in the base of the vesicle become infected with the viruses. These viruses multiply within them, while the roof of the vesicle degenerates, revealing an ulcer. Over the next few days this ulcer heals. We see this most often when someone has a cold sore, but the same thing occurs when the virus infects one of the sex organs.

It would seem that this is the end of the infection, but not so. As the viruses have been replicating inside the vesicle, many will have located the sensory endings of nerve cells. The viruses enter these cells and travel along the nerve fibers until they reach the nerve's main cell body, which is tucked next to the spinal cord. The viruses can then sit there inactive for years, simply waiting for a chance to become reactivated, travel back along the nerve, and establish a new outbreak of the disease. Once infected, most people experience four or five recurrences each year.

Region of operation

Genital herpes may not be deadly, but it can be physically painful, and emotionally debilitating. Estimates suggest that 20 percent of the American population—over 50 million people—are infected with genital herpes. Studies show that more than half a million Americans are diagnosed with genital herpes each year, and that the largest increase is occurring in young teens. The numbers of people affected in developing countries vary hugely depending on country, with some as low as two percent, and others as high as 75 percent. On top of this, there is evidence that people who are infected with herpes are at increased risk of additionally becoming infected with HIV if they have unprotected sex with an HIV-positive person.

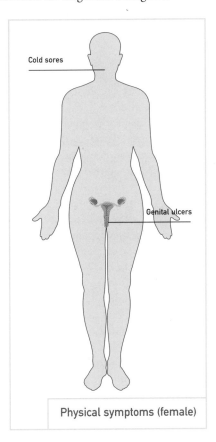

Cold sores

Genital ulcers

Physical symptoms (female)

Developments in treatment

In 1985, the first anti-viral drugs came onto the market and medicines were targeted at treating herpes. They work by preventing cells from building new copies of the viral genetic material. While this is a big step forward, there are signs that versions of the virus are emerging that can evade this drug—prevention is therefore still far better than cure.

Syphilis

Agent: bacterium
Treponema pallidum
First recorded: antiquity
Region: global

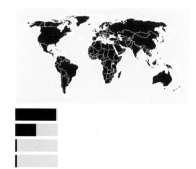

Infectivity	
Severity of illness	
Likelihood of dying if ill	
Bio-weapon threat	

T. pallidum was discovered as the underlying cause of syphilis in 1905, but the disease has been recognized for centuries. Historians have argued for years over whether fifteenth-century explorer Christopher Columbus and his crew brought this disease to Europe from the "New World," or whether the disease had always been there. Either way, it is certainly part of the disease scene now. People usually become infected through sexual activity with other infected individuals. The disease can also be passed from a mother to the fetus in her womb, or by the baby picking up the disease from the mucus that it encounters during birth. Rarely, syphilis has been acquired by transfusion of infected blood.

Symptoms and effects

If you don't treat it, syphilis becomes a progressive disease that moves through four different stages: primary, secondary, latent and tertiary. *T. pallidum* initially enters the body by burying into soft mucosal tissue or through damaged skin. Once inside, it rapidly enters the lymphatic system and spreads throughout the body. This bacterium is highly infectious, and as few as 10 organisms may be all that it takes to initiate an infection. The bacteria multiply at the initial entry site, and after an average incubation period of three weeks a painless bacteria-filled ulcer forms. These "chancres" are normally on the external genitalia, but may occur on the cervix, around the anus, or in the mouth. Kissing someone with mouth chancres is all it takes to pick up the disease. The chancre usually heals within three to six weeks, but then, between two and 12 weeks later, the symptoms of secondary syphilis develop: highly infectious ulcers break out almost anywhere on the body.

Slowly, these sores heal, but the bacteria don't go away—they just lie in wait. The person is in a latent phase of the disease, and relapses of secondary ulcers can occur at any time. Decades later, a person can develop tertiary syphilis. This is a slowly progressive, destructive inflammatory disease that can affect any organ; when it affects the brain victims gradually lose their sanity.

Region of operation

Syphilis thrives in social conditions where people have many sexual contacts. Health professionals who monitor sexual health have seen great changes in the numbers of men and women who become infected as different sexual practices become common in both heterosexual and homosexual communities. Currently, around 40,000 people in the U.S.A. are believed to have the disease, 80 percent of whom are African-Americans. In the U.K., the infection rate is low, but the country runs costly screening programs to ensure that the bacteria do not get into donated blood or blood products.

Developments in treatment

Being a bacterium, syphilis can be treated by antibiotics. In fact, treating soldiers during the Second World War was one of the first mass uses of these drugs. Controlling the disease involves making sure that all of an individual's sexual contacts are treated once one person is found to have the disease.

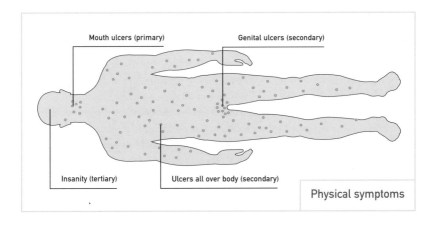

Mouth ulcers (primary) Genital ulcers (secondary)

Insanity (tertiary) Ulcers all over body (secondary)

Physical symptoms

Gonorrhea

Agent: bacterium
Nesseria gonorrhea
First recorded: 1879
Region: global

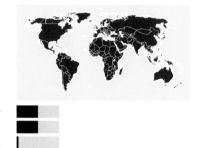

Infectivity	■
Severity of illness	■
Likelihood of dying if ill	▌
Bio-weapon threat	▌

Gonorrhea is a classical venereal disease, being spread almost exclusively by sexual promiscuity. It has a short incubation period, and is now relatively easy to diagnose and treat.

Origins

Gonorrhea has probably existed since pre-historic times and seems to have been described by Chinese writers more than 5,000 years ago. A disease that fits its description was also recorded by the ancient Arabs, Greeks, Indians, and Romans. The second-century Greek medic Galen named it in the mistaken belief that it was an involuntary flow of semen (*gono* means seed, *rhoia* means flux), but in 1879 Albert Neisser discovered the *gonococcus* bacterium.

Symptoms and effects

About 80 percent of infected women do not develop any symptoms, while only 10 percent of infected men are symptom-free. The most common symptom that causes people to seek medical help is when a man finds he has pain on passing urine. This normally comes a few days after having unprotected vaginal or anal sexual intercourse with an infected partner. The pain is often accompanied by a nasty and uncontrollable discharge from the penis. Most women seek treatment because they find that their partner is infected. If it is untreated in a woman, it can lead to widespread inflammation in her pelvic region, which in turn leads to her becoming infertile.

If the bacteria leave the sexual organs and start wandering around the body, they can cause a form of arthritis, fever, and pain in the joints.

Newborn infants can also catch the disease as they pick up mucus during their delivery. If this gets into their eyes and they are not treated, it can make them blind.

Region of operation

The rates of gonorrhea had been dropping significantly in the years up to the 1980s, but since then changing sexual practices in many countries have led to distinct increases. Figures for the U.K., for example, show a steady increase from around 10,000 cases in 1995 to 24,000 in 2005. In Israel, following a long period of decline from 40 per 100,000 in 1970 to 0.74 per 100,000 in 1997, rates began to increase in 1998, and by 2001 had reached 13.8 per 100,000. Most of the people with recorded infection are males aged 20-44 years, and there is a real danger of a large undetected rate of infection in young women.

Developments in treatment

Once the bacterium was isolated in 1879, doctors could start to think of ways of treating the disease. Before antibiotics arrived, one of the first treatments was to put silver nitrate in the eyes of newborn babies who were born to infected mothers. It went a long way to preventing blindness. Now, antibiotics can clear up the infection quickly, and if it hasn't been in the body long enough to cause long-term damage to internal organs, people should recover completely.

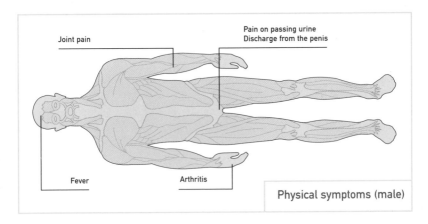

Joint pain

Pain on passing urine
Discharge from the penis

Fever

Arthritis

Physical symptoms (male)

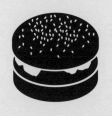

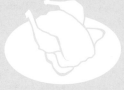

Part Four:

Food- and
Water-borne
Diseases

Salmonella

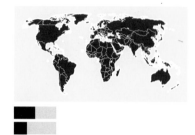

Agent: bacterium
Salmonella enterica
First recorded: antiquity
Region: global

Infectivity	
Severity of illness	
Likelihood of dying if ill	
Bio-weapon threat	

With a world population of around 6.5 billion, it is worrying that some 4.5 billion people suffer from some form of diarrheal disease each year. Many of these cases will be due to salmonella. To say someone has salmonella means they are ill, but it doesn't narrow down the exact type of bacterium that is troubling them very much. There are well over 2,000 different types of salmonella, and none of them is pleasant.

Origins

Even though people would have been falling to its power for centuries, salmonella was only named in 1900 by the French bacteriologist Joseph Lignieres in honor of American veterinary pathologist Daniel Salmon. While the boss took the fame, this particular form of bacterium had in fact been identified by Salmon's assistant, Theobald Smith.

Symptoms and effects

Salmonella is most associated with poultry and eggs, but in fact it can be contracted by eating any kind of undercooked food. Most types of salmonella cause a relatively short-lived form of diarrhea, but others can cause life-threatening illnesses. There are four broad sets of symptoms.

Enteric fever is one to avoid. *S. Typhi* or *S. Paratyphi* bury themselves into the lining of the gut and travel on into the lymph. This part of the body's plumbing gives them a free ride to the lymph nodes in the abdomen, and provides accommodation while they multiply and spill over into the bloodstream. Now the liver, gallbladder, spleen, kidney, and bone marrow become infected. Untreated, this phase can last for seven to ten days. The bacteria expand in great numbers within all these organs and then pour back into the blood, triggering a raging fever. The infected parts of the gut also start to die. Untreated, this classic typhoid fever kills one in five infected people. It is difficult to track within a population because it can either trigger illness within a few days of moving on board, or lie in wait for a couple of months.

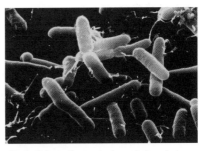

Above *Salmonella enterica* bacteria have hair-like appendages that help them to move.

Gastroenteritis is a second version, causing vomiting, fever, stomach cramps, and diarrhea. There are any number of *S. enterica* waiting to do this to you if you take them in as you eat or drink. The good news is that the bacteria this time stay inside the gut. You may be lucky and get away with a few bouts of loose stools—nothing too much to worry about. On the other hand, you could be laid up with an illness that involves frequently passing offensive watery, green stools, and in between times lying in bed shivering with a fever and stomach cramps. If you can't keep enough fluids in your body, your blood pressure can drop so much that your kidneys start to fail.

A so-called metastatic form of the disease is a third alternative. In this, the bacteria travel throughout the body, and then set up shop in various locations. These infections can cause damage to heart tissue, joints, and implanted medical devices; they can also leave the person with a form of arthritis.

The fourth option is to become a carrier. Here, the person shows no symptoms, but instead harbors the bacteria and deposits them daily in his or her stools. Fewer than one in 100 patients under the age of 20 become carriers after having the disease, but this can rise to 10 in 100 in older adults. At any age, women are twice as likely to become carriers as men.

Historic outbreaks
In Western countries, outbreaks of salmonella can often be linked to a restaurant where a member of staff was unwell, came to work, and didn't look

after their personal hygiene properly. Alternatively, not cooking food adequately can lead to problems. Over 300 people became ill after eating at a restaurant in Kershaw County, South Carolina, between May 19 and May 20, 2005. It appears that the turkey wasn't cooked thoroughly.

Developments in treatment

The treatment needed will depend on the type of disease that the bacteria are causing. In the case of enteric fever, rapid treatment with drugs like chloramphenicol or ciprofloxacin is essential. If the problem is gastroenteritis, keeping fluids and salts in the body can be all that is needed. If the bacteria are in the bloodstream, antibiotics need injecting there as well—and quickly.

Used as a weapon

To prove that bacteria are easy to use as a weapon, you need look no further than salmonella, then ask what happened in Oregon in 1984. An obscure religious sect called the Rajneeshees decided to try to influence an election, and their plan was to reduce the number of people going out to vote by ensuring that many of them were ill on the day. Their main action involved sprinkling salmonella-laden water over a salad bar in 10 of the local town's restaurants—700 people became ill. Suspicion fell on the sect only after they brought in bus-loads of homeless people and signed them up to vote.

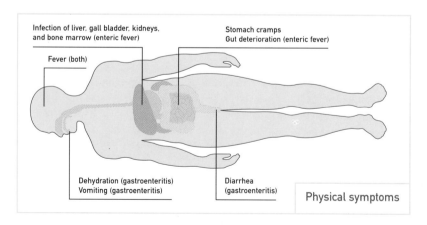

Infection of liver, gall bladder, kidneys, and bone marrow (enteric fever)

Stomach cramps
Gut deterioration (enteric fever)

Fever (both)

Dehydration (gastroenteritis)
Vomiting (gastroenteritis)

Diarrhea (gastroenteritis)

Physical symptoms

Cholera

Agent: bacterium
Vibrio cholerae (Family *Vibrionaceae*)
First recorded: 1563
Region: Africa, Asia, and Latin America

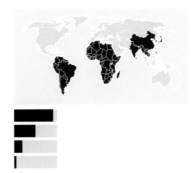

Infectivity	▉▉
Severity of illness	▉
Likelihood of dying if il	▉
Bio-weapon threat	▏

Of all the water-borne infections, cholera has a reputation for aggression—and it is one that is deserved. Cholera can kill in 24 hours. In recorded history, it has swept around the world in seven distinct and devastating pandemics, and the seventh is reluctant to go away.

Origins
Throughout history, populations all over the world have had outbreaks of a disease that fits the description of cholera. Ancient Sanskrit writings from 500 to 400 B.C.E. record a disease that sounds like cholera in India, although a 1563 epidemic described in a report from India is the first clear record of the disease. By the nineteenth century, cholera had spread from the Orient to other parts of the world.

Symptoms and effects
People become infected by drinking water or eating food contaminated by *Vibrio cholerae* bacteria. The bacteria live in the gut of an infected person and are passed on in their feces. Once the bacteria are around, infection of others becomes almost inevitable if sanitation is poor, or people don't look after their personal and domestic hygiene.

Symptoms include the sudden onset of effortless and uncontrollable stools that have the consistency of rice water. Vomiting may also occur. The massive loss of fluid from the body means that the victims rapidly dehydrate. Blood pressure falls, cramps develop in the patient's legs and abdomen, and then their temperature falls as their organs start to fail. Death can occur within 24

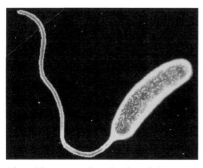

Above The comma-shaped *Vibrio cholerae* bacterium uses its "tail" to move.

hours of the first symptoms if you don't get prompt medical treatment.

It is, however, possible to be infected and show no symptoms. Alternatively, some people get ill and recover, but still harbor low levels of the bug in their gut. Such symptom-less carriers excrete *vibrio* bacteria every now and again for anything up to 15 months.

Historic outbreaks

Cholera thrives in situations where civil sanitation breaks down. This can be due to conflict or calamity. On August 2, 1885 a massive rain-storm hit Chicago. The drains were overwhelmed, and raw sewage flooded the streets and poured into the lake that supplied the city with its drinking water. More than 80,000 people died.

This is the key reason for having two separate sets of drains in towns and cities. One carries sewage and runs at a more or less constant rate whatever the weather. The other is devoted to carrying rain water. These can be empty for much of the year, but then instantly fill after a heavy downpour, carrying the water safely away, and preventing it from flushing raw sewage into the waterways.

Since 1817, health watchers have recorded seven distinct pandemics of cholera. The first six originated in the Ganges Delta of India, but the seventh began in Indonesia in 1961. This pandemic has now spread the El Tor 01 biotype of the bacterium throughout the world, probably carried in the ballast water of supertankers. It has caused large-scale background levels of infection in many countries, and as such has pretty well moved from being a pandemic to being endemic—it is effectively just a part of the natural environment. There is now a fear that an eighth pandemic is starting. Variant *V. cholerae* 0139 has spread around Asia—it is now present in 11 countries—and seems to have no desire to go away. What's more, having an immunity to other forms of cholera does not protect you from this one.

Developments in treatment

Fluid and salts are the keys to survival. There is nothing particularly technical about it, as long as you have a way of making sure that the fluid is clean. Oral rehydration therapy is based around dissolving a tablespoon of sugar and a teaspoon of salt in a pint of water, then drinking it.

Various antibiotics can reduce the time for which a person will shed viruses into the sewer, and therefore reduce the chance of passing the disease on. The only problem here is that it will inevitably lead to a generation of antibiotic-resistant versions of the bacteria, so many health professionals question whether it is worth using in all but the most extreme situations.

Developing vaccines has proved to be difficult because a vaccine can be targeted at only one version of the bacterium, and there are over 100 versions out there.

Used as a weapon

The Geneva Convention prohibits any deliberate contamination of water. In war, however, water often becomes contaminated when a community's infrastructure is hit. Bombing roads or bridges will inevitably disrupt the services that run alongside them, which risks triggering an outbreak of this disease. The cynic would suggest that some war planners will be aware of this, and be only too keen to take advantage of it.

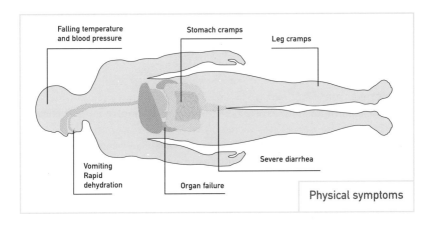

Falling temperature and blood pressure

Stomach cramps

Leg cramps

Vomiting
Rapid dehydration

Organ failure

Severe diarrhea

Physical symptoms

Polio

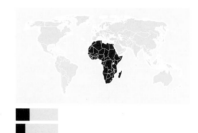

Agent: Virus (Family: *Picornaviridae*)
Poliovirus (3 types)
First recorded: antiquity
Region: almost eradicated

Infectivity	■
Severity of illnes	■
Likelihood of dying if ill	I
Bio-weapon threat	■■■■

There is the possibility that polio viruses could join the short list of successes in disease eradication, which currently contains only one entry—smallpox. In 1988, the World Health Organization launched its Global Polio Eradication Initiative (G.P.E.I.), with the aim of sweeping the disease into obscurity by the end of the millennium. The timetable may have slipped, but the goal is getting tantalizingly close—the number of annual diagnosed cases has been reduced from the hundreds of thousands to around a thousand.

Origins

Polio is an ancient disease and its effects have been known since prehistory. There are Egyptian paintings and carvings that show otherwise healthy people with withered limbs, or children walking with a cane, and one theory has it that the Roman Emperor Claudius contracted the disease as a child, causing him to walk with a limp for the rest of his life. However, the first medical report on polio was by Jakob Heine in 1840.

Symptoms and effects

Three versions of the virus exist and all can trigger any one of three different versions of the disease.

The vast majority of people show no symptoms of an infection, excrete the virus in their stools, and gain immunity—so far, so good. A few get a headache, stiff neck, and back pain as they develop viral meningitis. This goes away within a few days—again, not too dangerous. About one in 1,000 children, or one in 75 adults, who become infected develop the paralytic form of the disease. These people go through an initial infection phase of fever, sore throat, nausea, and headaches, which lasts around five to seven days, and then seem to get better. During this stage, the virus has been ingested with food or water, been absorbed in the gut, and multiplied itself in lymph nodes in the abdomen. The fever occurred when viral particles flooded from the nodes and migrated in the bloodstream to the central nervous system.

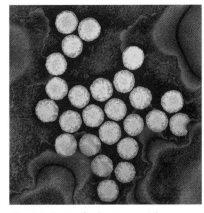

Above A cluster of polio virus particles.

After three to five days of apparent recovery, the second phase starts. The muscles become paralyzed as the virus destroys some nerves and causes others to become inflamed. The destroyed nerves are seldom replaced, so the paralysis is permanent. Any nerves that simply became inflamed can recover over a few months, and so the muscles they control regain most of their function.

Region of operation

In 1988 there were over 350,000 reported cases in 125 countries, with 1,000 children becoming paralyzed each day. However, by 2003 the count had dropped to 784 recorded cases worldwide. The disease was now only to be found lurking in Nigeria, Niger, Egypt, Pakistan, Afghanistan, and India.

Political unrest and suspicion, however, can damage the best-laid plans. In 2003, rumors spread in northern Nigeria that the polio vaccine was laced with HIV and also contained a contraceptive. Fear spread that this was part of an anti-Islamic plot, and uptake of the vaccine plummeted. This meant that many people, including newborn children, were left vulnerable.

During the eleven-month boycott, the disease spread across Africa, from Guinea on the Atlantic to Sudan on the Red Sea. As cases started to rise, travelers inadvertently shipped it to twenty-one countries that had previously become polio-free. Disease fighters set to work and, by 2006, were basically back to where they had been at the turn of the millennium—but more than ever aware that committing polio to history was not going to be simple.

Developments in treatment

One of the overarching problems in this endgame has been the nature of the vaccine. Until recently, the only option was one that gave people a dose of a modified, live virus. The problem here was that children given the vaccine excreted large quantities of virus in their feces, and could potentially infect other non-vaccinated people. This is not good news if you ever intend to phase vaccination out.

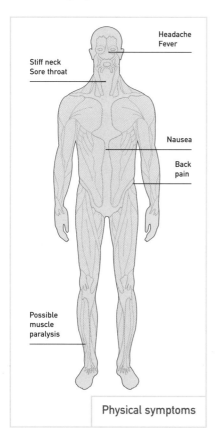

Headache
Fever

Stiff neck
Sore throat

Nausea

Back
pain

Possible
muscle
paralysis

Physical symptoms

Another problem with this vaccine is that it can lead to outbreaks of the virus. This has occured as recently as August 2006 in China, although it is very rare, and tends to occur in areas where there is low take-up of the vaccine.

However, in 2006 an alternative vaccine became available. While it only targets one strain of the virus at a time, it is not excreted. This means that it needs to be used more carefully, but provides a way of protecting people without fearing that you could re-seed the bug.

Used as a weapon

Many countries are now withdrawing their polio vaccination programs in the belief that the disease has been eradicated. However, this leaves people vulnerable to a deliberate, terror-driven attempt to re-introduce it.

Transmissible Spongiform Encephalopathies

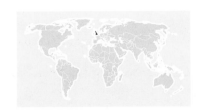

Agent: prion
Proteinaceous infectious particle (prion)
First recorded: vCJD appeared in 1996
Region: UK

Infectivity	
Severity of illness	
Likelihood of dying if ill	
Bio-weapon threat	

There is a simple dogma when it comes to infectious disease. First, it needs an infectious agent—some bug that can move into an individual and trigger the illness. This separates it from something like skin cancer, which you cannot catch from another person because there is no agent that can move from one person to another. Second, this agent must be capable of building new copies of itself, so that once it has infected one person, it can multiply and move on. Third, in order to perform this feat of replication it must come with the genetic instructions that order the construction process.

Transmissible spongiform encephalopathies have been an enigma for years because, search as they can, no one has found a particle that fulfills all of these three points. It would appear that these diseases have broken the basic rules of infection; the best guess at the moment is that the infective particle is a simple lump of protein. What is more curious is that it is a variant of a protein that is normally found in the body. However, it appears that once your body has absorbed this misshapen molecule, some as yet unknown process sets about multiplying it—and the result is biological chaos.

Origins

For human beings, things started to become critical in November 1986, when a disturbing disease broke out among cattle in the U.K. The cows seemed to

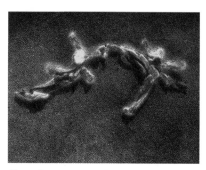

Above Scrapie-associated protein strands taken from the brain of an infected hamster.

be losing control of their bodies, and "Mad Cow Disease" entered the newspaper headlines. It wasn't long before this disease was linked to a similar condition in sheep and goats known to farmers as "scrapie." Scientists soon concluded that the cattle had caught the disease because brains from scrapie-affected sheep had been incorporated into their feed. "Don't worry," said the politicians, "this can't jump to humans." All the same, a large-scale eradication plan was launched to rid the U.K. of affected animals.

Then, in spring 1996, came the announcement that humans could pick up the disease. Panic broke out. Beef sales crashed, and some predictions suggested that tens of thousands of people could die. A decade later, policy makers started to calm down, but not before a massive slaughter program had cleaned up the U.K. herd. Very few people had in fact come down with the disease—was the disease really a threat in the first place, or had the threat been averted by rapid and decisive action?

Symptoms and effects

As the disease was similar to a rare brain disease called Creutzfeldt-Jakob disease (CJD), it was named "variant CJD" or vCJD. It is a rapid degenerative illness that normally kills people within a year of their first symptoms.

At first, it appears that victims "simply" have depression, but soon they develop coordination problems, memory loss, and mood swings. Then come pins and needles, pains in the limbs, bad headaches, rashes, and short-term memory loss. It isn't long before they are visiting a neurologist. With no treatment available, medics and family can only look on as the disease destroys the person's brain, and they die.

As of 2004, 157 people worldwide have acquired and died of vCJD; 148 of these deaths have been in the United Kingdom. People are still being diagnosed with the disease, but the number of new cases currently seems to be dropping. However, due to the long incubation period for prion diseases—years or even decades—the full extent of the human vCJD epidemic is still not fully known.

Developments in treatment
It is often hard enough to devise therapies for treatments that are clearly understood, but developing a treatment for a disease we don't understand is almost impossible. Some doctors have tried using the anti-malarial drug quinacrine and the anti-psychotic chloropromazine, but have not produced any real results. A few have claimed that injecting the anti-blood-clotting drug pentosan polysulphate directly into the spaces around the brain can help, but there is no real evidence of substantial benefit. One trial had a go with the brain-cell-protecting drug flupirtine: patients showed marginally improved abilities to think, but the effect was short-lived as it didn't improve survival.

Potential threat to civilization
This may not have threatened our civilization, but it should warn us that extreme forms of agriculture can create unusual problems, and for many farmers it was the end of the herd that their family had built up over centuries. It also serves as a reminder that we can never be sure that we fully understand infectious disease— biology can always conjure up new possibilities.

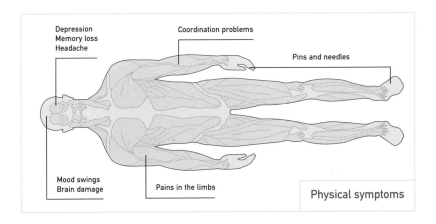

Depression
Memory loss
Headache

Coordination problems

Pins and needles

Mood swings
Brain damage

Pains in the limbs

Physical symptoms

Hepatitis A

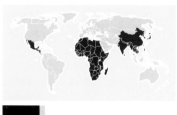

Agent: virus
Hepatitis A virus (HAV)
First recorded: 1960s
Region: Africa, Asia, and Central America

Infectivity	
Severity of illness	
Likelihood of dying if ill	
Bio-weapon threat	

Assumed to be an ancient disease, the viruses that cause a range of liver diseases were only identified in the 1960s and 1970s. The first to be identified was rather unimaginatively called hepatitis A virus, or HAV for short.

Origins

This virus leaves an infected person in their feces and moves on as a second person puts it in their mouth, a method called fecal–oral transmission. Good personal hygiene is therefore rather important, particularly if you happen to be changing the diaper of a child whom you know to be infected.

Most people, however, catch it from contaminated water. Alternatively, you can pick it up from eating fruit or salad vegetables that have been watered with contaminated water and then not washed clean, or washed with unclean water. Therefore, a basic rule for travelers in highly affected areas is not to eat food that hasn't been cooked, and that has preferably been cooked recently.

Raw seafood that has been harvested from contaminated coastal waters is another carrier. Seafood feeds by sifting vast quantities of water, and if the virus is around, some of it will stick. Again, cooking it will help protect you.

Symptoms and effects

This is a very common virus in humans, but one that does not usually kill. If you pick it up, it will take somewhere between 15 and 50 days before the virus sets to work, although most cases appear within 28 days. You may show no symptoms. Alternatively, you could get a combination of yellow eyes and dark urine. You could also feel very sick, have a fever, and be tired. Add to this a stomach ache and possible vomiting, and it is hardly surprising that you could also lose your appetite. Symptoms last for anywhere between two and six months, after which you will be immune to it should you ever encounter the virus again.

Each year about 150 million people around the world develop symptoms. However, this is only the tip of an epidemic iceberg as many more become infected without developing symptoms. Infants younger than six months seldom show any signs of the virus, and are therefore perfect vehicles for silently transporting the disease from one person to another.

Developments in treatment

A vaccine was developed in the 1970s. It is created by exposing viruses to formaldehyde. This damages them enough to prevent them from causing disease, but when they are injected the body spots them and learns how to destroy them. Next time the body sees a virulent version, it is ready to pounce.

Short-term protection can be gained by having injections of gamma globulin, a protein that plays a key role in fighting infections. It gives a general boost to your immune system and, depending on which version you take, can give a measure of protection from between six months and ten years.

However, once again, the most important advance in treatment throughout the world is the provision of clean water.

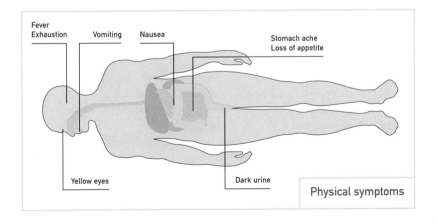

Physical symptoms

Botulism

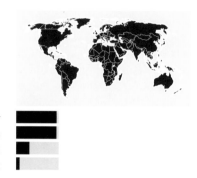

Agent: bacterium
Clostridium botulinum
First recorded: 1793
Region: global, particularly Alaska

Infectivity	████
Severity of illness	████
Likelihood of dying if ill	██
Bio-weapon threat	█

It's not the bacteria you need to be worried about with botulism—a rare but serious paralytic illness—it's the toxin that the bacteria produce. One of the deadliest chemicals known to man, botulin blocks nerve function and leads to respiratory and musculoskeletal paralysis.

Origins

In Wildbad, Germany in 1793, an outbreak of disease suddenly confined 13 people to their beds and killed six of them. They had all eaten a locally produced blood sausage. Over the next few years, local health officer Justinius Kerner recorded 230 similar cases. All of the people had consumed similar sausages, so he named the disease using the Latin word for sausage—botulus.

Then, in 1895, in the small Belgian town of Ellezelles, an outbreak occurred among thirty-four musicians who had shared a raw ham preserved in salt brine. Twenty-three of the musicians became sick and three died. Emile van Ermengem, Professor of Microbiology at the University of Ghent, investigated the incident and discovered that the root cause was a spore-forming bacterium that grew only in places where there was no oxygen—in scientific jargon, it was an "obligate anaerobe." This bacterium we now know as *Clostridium botulinum*.

It is *C. botulinum*'s ability to survive in the open as spores, combined with its ability to thrive in zones that have no oxygen, that makes it such a stealthy foe. Communities that traditionally consume foods preserved by fermentation are at particular risk, and anyone who bottles or cans fruit at home needs to take care not to let this killer get to the table.

What happens is that *C. botulinum*'s spores get into the food mix before the container is sealed for storage. The food is preserved either by heating or pickling, but if the heat is not sufficient, or the fermentation is too slow, the spores germinate and the bacteria will thrive in this airless condition. As they grow, the bacteria release a toxin, and even if the organisms die before you eat the food, the toxin will still get you.

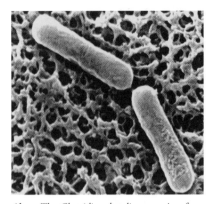

Above The *Clostridium botulinum* species of bacteria, which grows in badly preserved canned goods, can cause serious food poisoning in humans.

The good news is that the toxin is easily destroyed by heating, so cook the preserved food and you will be safe. It is also very unusual for anyone to become infected with this species of bacteria, because there is too much oxygen around in the body, which means the human body is not a natural home for the bacteria.

Although the most common way of contracting the illness is through eating food contaminated with the botulism toxin, it can also be caused by consuming the spores of the botulinum bacteria, which then grow in the intestines and release a toxin (infant botulism) or through a wound becoming infected with *C. botulinum* (wound botulism—the rarest form of the illness).

Symptoms and effects

The symptoms usually appear within 12 to 36 hours of eating the toxin, but they can appear as early as 6 hours or as late as 10 days after consuming it. People become weak, suffer from vertigo, and get blurred or double vision and a dry mouth. Soon, they have difficulty swallowing and their speech becomes slurred. Their neck and arms can become weak, and they may start to vomit and develop severe diarrhea or constipation. Victims do not develop a fever, but a paralysis of their chest muscles makes it increasingly difficult to breathe. These are all symptoms of the muscle paralysis caused by the bacterial toxin. If left untreated, these symptoms may progress to cause paralysis of the arms, legs, trunk, respiratory muscles, and in some cases, eventually death.

Developments in treatment

In the past fifty years, improvements in the supportive care given to patients with botulism have led to a fall in the fatality rate from around 50 percent to 8 percent. An antitoxin, which blocks the action of the toxin circulating in the blood, does also exist. If you are diagnosed early and take the antitoxin in time, your chance of recovery increases greatly. Even so, recovery may take weeks until your muscles have thrown the toxin out and can operate again. The breathing difficulties and paralysis that occur with severe botulism can require a breathing machine and several months worth of intensive medical and nursing care. Also, as each case of botulism is a potential public health emergency, it is vital that the authorities identify the source of the outbreak and ensure that no contaminated food remains.

The main development in the botulism story is in the fashion industry, where the toxin is now used as "Botox" to paralyze muscles in the face and iron out wrinkles. If you decide to have this treatment, it is worth remembering that you are injecting one of the most potent poisons known to man, and on a few occasions even small quantities of the toxin have left people feeling generally weak and unwell.

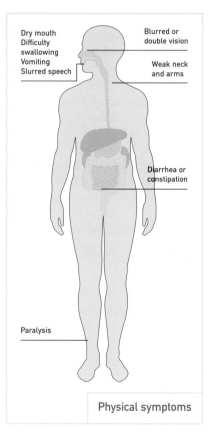

Dry mouth
Difficulty swallowing
Vomiting
Slurred speech

Blurred or double vision

Weak neck and arms

Diarrhea or constipation

Paralysis

Physical symptoms

E. coli O157: H7

Agent: bacterium
Escherich coli
First recorded: 1885
Region: global

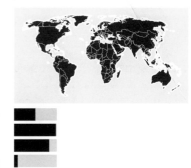

Infectivity	
Severity of illness	
Likelihood of dying if ill	
Bio-weapon threat	

As you sit there reading this, your gut will be packed with millions upon millions of *E. coli*. Hopefully, the ones you have are the friendly variety, which are welcomed into the body because they play a vital role in digestion. However, there are a few varieties of this particular species that play nasty, and *E. coli* O157:H7 has got a particularly bad name for itself.

Origins

German pediatrician and bacteriologist Theodor Escherich was the first person to identify this type of bacterium when studying the contents of the human colon in 1885. He called them *Bacterium coli*, but the name was later changed to recognise his achievement. It didn't take long before Escherich realized that various strains of *E. coli* were responsible for diarrhea in infants and gastroenteritis in adults. Because it grows so well in a laboratory, it has also become one of the most studied bacteria on earth.

The variant *E. coli* O157:H7 was first recognized as a cause of illness in the U.S.A. in 1982 during an outbreak of severe bloody diarrhea, which was traced to a batch of contaminated hamburgers. Now that laboratories are looking for this particular strain, pathologists have discovered that it is the cause of a couple of distinctive diseases.

Symptoms and effects

While other forms of *E. coli* can cause meningitis in children, *E. coli* O157:H7 is much more likely to attack the gut and kidneys, and in some cases can cause kidney failure. Its main weapon is a protein that scientists

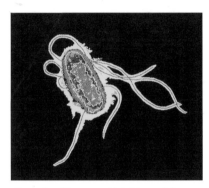

Above *E. coli* is a normal inhabitant of the human intestine and is usually harmless, but under certain conditions its numbers may increase and cause infection.

recognize because it kills Vero cells (cells from monkey kidneys). This toxin is also pretty destructive within the human body.

Thus, *E. coli* is yet another organism that causes the person to have abdominal cramps and severe, acute diarrhea, but this time the stool is colored red. This is because the toxins from the bacteria have done so much damage to the gut's lining that it is bleeding—this is called "hemorrhagic colitis."

If the bacteria break through from the gut into the body, you can move on to "hemolytic uremic syndrome." In this case, the person's kidneys soon fail, red and white blood cells die, and the victim develops a fever. This complication occurs in two to seven percent of *E. coli* infections and is most common in children under the age of five or the elderly. One in ten of these people will also develop a respiratory infection. Between five and fifteen out of 100 die.

Historic outbreaks

This illness is often called "hamburger disease," because the bacteria are often introduced to a person in poorly-cooked ground beef. When not living in humans, it hides in cattle, so can be transferred to meat during the slaughtering and butchering process. This is a particular problem with hamburger meat, as the grinding process mixes the organism thoroughly into the meat. Unpasteurized fruit juices have also proved to be popular places for the bacteria to lurk. The illness can also be passed from person to person, so poor hygiene is a key factor in spreading the illness. Infection can also occur after drinking unpasteurized milk if the bacteria was present on the cow's udders or farm equipment, or by swimming in or drinking contaminated water. Although scientists do not yet know how many bacteria are needed to cause disease, it is suspected to be very small.

The scale of the problem can be seen by looking at one of the world's biggest consumers of meat, the U.S.A., where over 73,000 people become ill due to *E. coli* O157 each year. Over 2,000 of these people end up in hospital, and 60 or so die. If you look wider, the issue gets bigger. *E. coli* in its various forms is one of the agents that causes 3 million children in the developing world to die of diarrhea each year.

When it goes wrong, it can go very wrong. In the middle of July 1996, a massive outbreak occurred among elementary school children in the city of Sakai, Japan. School meals in the city had been contaminated by *E. coli* O157, and 12,680 people developed symptoms of the disease. Of these, 121 cases developed hemolytic uremic syndrome, and three girls died.

Developments in treatment

Most people recover without antibiotics or any other specific treatment within five to ten days. Antibiotics can help people with severe symptoms to fight the disease, but there is no vaccine currently on the market.

As with many food-borne diseases, prevention is better than cure. Good hygiene is important, as is ensuring that you cook ground beef thoroughly before eating. Avoiding unpasteurized milk and juice can also help.

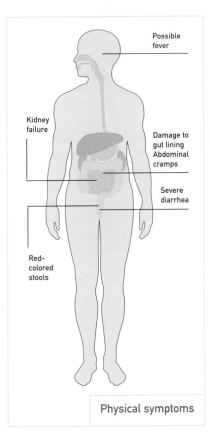

Possible fever

Kidney failure

Damage to gut lining
Abdominal cramps

Severe diarrhea

Red-colored stools

Physical symptoms

Giardia

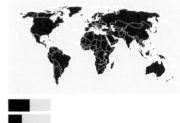

Agent: Protozoa
Giardia lamblia (or *Giardia intestinalis*)
First recorded: 1859
Region: global

Infectivity	
Severity of illness	
Likelihood of dying if ill	
Bio-weapon threat	

Protozoa are single-celled animals that tend to live by eating bacteria. Some manage to live alongside us and within us without causing any problems, but many others create problems. *Giardia lamblia* can do both.

Origins

Like a number of micro-organisms, *G. lamblia* can form cysts. These egg-like capsules enable the organism to lie dormant for long periods of time, waiting for the chance to move into a new environment where it might thrive. These cysts are robust, and will withstand quite high levels of chlorination, so can, on occasion, get through the cleaning systems used in domestic water supplies. A key way of keeping bugs like this out of our drinking water is to keep animals and humans out of our reservoirs, because if they are infected and swim there they may leave behind an unwanted gift that is difficult to remove.

Symptoms and effects

The giardia parasite lives in vast quantities in the intestines of infected humans or animals. A single bowel movement will release millions of the protozoa, and these are normally picked up by taking in water that has become contaminated. This water can be in a swimming pool, hot tub, lake, river, or pond, or even in a public drinking water supply if something has gone wrong.

Alongside diarrhea and stomach cramps, giardiosis tends to create stools that are greasy and float. This is because the protozoa disrupt the way in which fats are absorbed in the gut, and it also generates a lot of gas—stools are consequently full of fat and gas. The diarrhea and inability to absorb fat may cause a person to lose weight and become dehydrated, and the symptoms can last for six weeks or longer.

Historic outbreaks

Traveling in parts of the world with poor water treatment always puts you at risk of picking up this infection, as in many parts of the developing world it is just part of the ecosystem. Developed countries are also riddled with it. Some surveys suggest that 20 to 30 percent of people working in day-care centers for elderly people harbor the disease without having symptoms. There are also occasional outbreaks. In June 1997, 100 people who had stayed at a campsite in Oregon became ill after drinking water from a system that combined groundwater from an untreated well with water from a chlorinated spring. A larger outbreak occurred in the town of Bergen, Norway, in the winter of 2004–2005. Over 1,000 people became ill as they drank water that had originally been drawn from the local lake. Local chlorination systems hadn't removed the cysts.

Developments in treatment

Antibiotics such as albenzazole, metronidazole, or furizolidone are often prescribed by doctors to treat giardiosis. However, some people may recover on their own without medication.

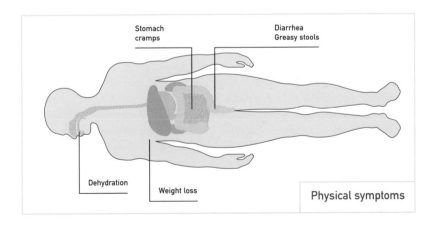

Stomach cramps

Diarrhea
Greasy stools

Dehydration

Weight loss

Physical symptoms

Listeria

Agent: bacterium
Listeria monocytogenes
First recorded: 1929
Region: global

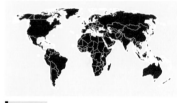

Infectivity	
Severity of illness	
Likelihood of dying if ill	
Bio-weapon threat	

If you are not a newborn baby or pregnant, this germ will probably pass you by. If you are, you need to actively avoid it.

Origins
The first recorded case of a human being infected with *L. monocytogenes* was in 1929, but it took until the early 1980s before we realized that it got to us in our food. Chilled, pre-cooked food is a wonderful environment for listeria, and the bug can also live well in unpasteurized foods, such as specialty cheeses. The risk increases if you are casual about use-by dates or damaged packaging.

Symptoms and effects
Infections in pregnant women are rare before about 20 weeks of pregnancy. After that, an infection will trigger mild chills, fever, and back pain. The woman may have a sore throat, headache, and occasionally has a eye infection and diarrhea. Quite frequently, there are no noticeable symptoms, but infections during pregnancy can lead to miscarriage, premature delivery, or stillbirth. If the child is born alive, there is a risk of the baby picking up the infection either in the womb or during the delivery, and between 30 and 60 percent of these babies die. If young babies pick up the infection a week or more after birth, the chances of dying falls to around 10 percent.

Over one month old, the only people susceptible to listeria are those whose immune system is not working well. These are often people taking immuno-suppressants to stop their body rejecting a transplant, people with HIV/AIDS, people on high doses of steroids, or those having treatment for cancer.

Region of operation

Since its discovery, cases of listeria have been reported across the globe. By 1986 over 1,800 cases a year were showing up in the U.S.A. alone, with more than 400 of these people dying.

Historic outbreaks

The bacteria can cause industrial as well as personal chaos. On October 9, 2002, Wampler Foods in Philadelphia recalled 295,000 pounds (134,000 kg) of ready-to-eat turkey and chicken products after a strain of *L. monocytogenes* was found in some of the products. A few days later, they expanded the recall to the 27.4 million pounds (12.4 million kg) of food that it had produced and released between May 1 and October 11 that year.

Developments in treatment

There is little agreement as to which is the best way to treat this disease, though many antibiotics seem to be good at clearing the bacteria out.

Potential threat to civilization

It may not threaten civilization, but listeria does serve as a reminder that, in a world of ever-more processed and ready-prepared meals, we need to act with ever-more vigilance. If we are casual, convenience foods will come at a cost.

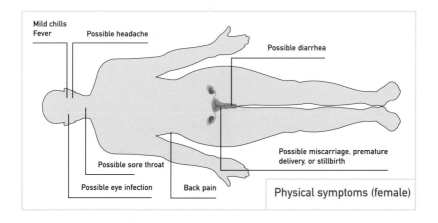

Mild chills
Fever
Possible headache
Possible diarrhea
Possible sore throat
Possible miscarriage, premature delivery, or stillbirth
Possible eye infection
Back pain
Physical symptoms (female)

Norwalk Virus

Agent: virus (Family *Calcivirus*)
Norwalk-like viruses
First recorded: 1972
Region: global

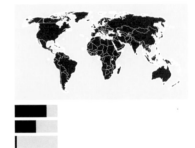

Infectivity	
Severity of illness	
Likelihood of dying if ill	
Bio-weapon threat	

Origins
First identified in 1972 when it showed up in Norwalk, Ohio, this virus appears to infect humans only. Again, it is passed on in stools, and poor hygiene, or consuming contaminated shellfish, are the main causes of outbreaks. When traveling in countries with poorly developed infrastructures, beware of ice and salads that have been prepared using local water.

Symptoms and effects
Norwalk brings with it the usual range of symptoms for gastroenteritis—nausea, vomiting, diarrhea, and stomach cramps. Most people will get better within three to five days, but a few will need to move into hospital and go on a drip to restore the levels of fluids in their body. It's unlikely to kill you, but for a few days you can feel distinctly ill.

Region of operation
Close-packed populations of people who do not keep up their guard properly are terrific places for Norwalk to operate. Schools are wonderful breeding grounds, as are entertainment facilities such as cruise liners that pack large numbers of people into small places and keep them that way for a few days.

Historic outbreaks
As passengers set out on a cruise liner, most intend to forget about all of life's worries, lie back, and rest for a week or so in the lap of luxury. Increasingly, however, this floating heaven has lost some of its pleasure as, one after another,

members of crew and passengers succumb to a Norwalk virus. For example, in July 2002 cruise organization Holland America had to take its ship *Ryndham* out of service for a few days to sanitize it after 388 of its passengers fell ill on an Alaskan cruise. In November of the same year, the same company found itself scrubbing down the *Amsterdam* after 500 people caught the virus on four separate voyages. A few days later, Disney found itself working hard to get their liner *Magic* back into service after 60 passengers fell ill. The worrying thing for the company was that the ship had only just come back into service after being thoroughly cleaned, due to 275 passengers catching Norwalk on a previous cruise.

Developments in treatment

As it is a virus, there are very few ways of tackling the disease, so the key way of breaking a chain of infection is to act responsibly. If you have it, keep to yourself for a few days. If your kids have it, keep them off school until they are well and truly clear. As a guideline, you should have stopped passing on the virus if you haven't been sick or had diarrhea for 48 hours.

Used as a weapon

As with any highly contagious disease, if you wanted to create a campaign of mild terror and great disruption, Norwalk would be a simple agent to use. However, the fact that it seldom kills would make it a low-level threat.

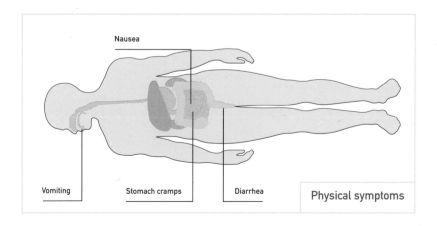

Nausea

Vomiting   Stomach cramps   Diarrhea   Physical symptoms

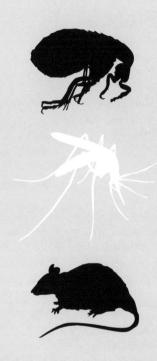

Part Five:

Animal-borne Diseases

Plague

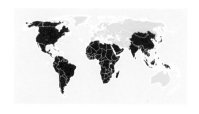

Agent: bacterium and flea
Yersinia pestis
First recorded: 1300s
Region: North and South America,
Africa, and Asia

Infectivity	
Severity of illness	
Likelihood of dying if ill	
Bio-weapon threat	

Historians estimate that in 1347 around 75 million people lived in Europe. By 1352, only five years later, the figure had dropped to 50 million. The cause was plague, or the "Black Death," so-called because of the blackening of the victim's skin. Almost simultaneous epidemics occurred across large portions of Asia and the Middle East in the same period, with this multi-regional pandemic causing at least 75 million deaths. The same disease is thought to have returned to Europe every generation until the 1700s, including the Great Plague of London in 1665–1666—one of the last great European outbreaks of the disease.

At the time of the first outbreak, no one realized that the agent of destruction was a bacterium carried by fleas that lived on rats. When outbreaks occurred, people tried to avoid contact with other people, but they were much less concerned about the rodents.

Origins

In the early 1330s plague broke out in China, and because China was linked to the rest of world through trade, the disease spread quickly—transported by rats hidden as stowaways among the cargo. When it got to the edge of the Black Sea, it infected an army that was besieging a city. In 1347, the army started dying, while those in the city remained unaffected—that is, until the besieging army started lobbing disease-ridden corpses over the walls. Soon, plague was at large in the city, and its occupants fled in ships. When the vessels arrived in Sicily in southern Italy, the few people left alive were surrounded by corpses, and the ports prevented them from leaving the ship. Sadly, they didn't stop the rats that ran ashore along the mooring ropes, and plague entered the country. As Italy had trade links with many other countries, it wasn't long before plague had spread across Western Europe.

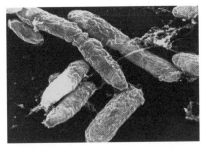

Above The *Yersinia pestis* bacteria, carried by the fleas on rats, is transferred to people when the fleas feed on human blood.

Plague left Europe in the seventeenth century as the black rat, which often lives in human dwellings, was replaced by the brown rat, which prefers to live in sewers. The last notable outbreak was in Moscow in 1771. The disease was completely eradicated in Europe only at the beginning of the nineteenth century, but it is still a threat in many different parts of the world, including areas of Africa, Asia, and the Americas—including the U.S.A.

Symptoms and effects

Y. pestis bacteria are transmitted from animal to animal and from animal to people by fleas. The fleas thrive in cool, humid weather, but die back in hot, dry weather, so you need to watch out if you are in endemic areas at the wrong time of year.

When a flea feeds on an infected animal, it draws in bacteria. These multiply and block the flea's gut. When the flea moves to a new animal, which this time could be a human, and feeds again, the blockage in its gut causes it to regurgitate some of its stomach contents. Bacteria from the gut therefore flood into the new host's bloodstream. The fleas are just as happy living on the backs of domestic cats as on rats, so these can be a problem in areas of the world where the disease is at large. The sputum of an infected person is also packed with bacteria, giving it another way of moving around.

Three different categories of illness can occur. In bubonic plague, which was the most commonly seen form of the disease during the Black Death, the insect bite causes a local infection that spreads to nearby lymph nodes in the neck, armpits, or groin. These "buboes" swell, then the bacteria start to spread through the body. Other symptoms include fever, headache, nausea, vomiting and aching joints. Without antibiotics, half of these people will die.

A person can also become infected by inhaling the bacteria. This pneumonic plague causes blood-pink sputum that can easily pass on the disease to others when the infected person coughs. It kills almost all people, unless it is treated very early.

In septicemic plague, the bacteria move into the bloodstream after arriving via either a bite or an inhaled aerosol. The shock of having so many bacteria flooding into the blood kills most people, even if they get treatment.

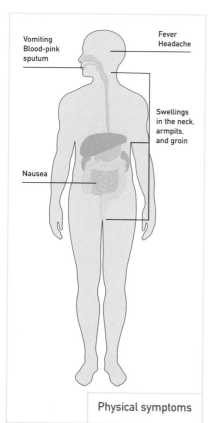

Physical symptoms

Developments in treatment

Given that plague has affected the outcome of major wars and has ravaged entire populations, it is intriguing to try to guess what the world would look like if antibiotics had been discovered 1,000 years earlier. Now that they are here, they reduce most of the cases of this disease to something that is relatively easy to treat.

Used as a weapon

Plague has been used in the past as a weapon, and could potentially be used as an agent of terror—imagine what the headline "Plague-infested rats released in New York" would do for the U.S. tourist industry.

Yellow Fever

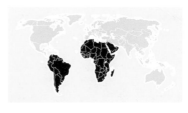

Agent: virus + mosquito
Flavivirus
(Family: *Flaviviridae*)
First recorded: 1648
Region: tropical South America and Africa

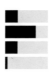

Infectivity	
Severity of illness	
Likelihood of dying if ill	
Bio-weapon threat	

Arthropod-borne viruses, or "arbo" viruses for short, come in many shapes and sizes, and over 500 have been documented so far. Yellow fever is one of the diseases that can result.

Currently, only around 250 people a year are recorded as having this disease, of whom around 70 die. However, health officials are fairly certain that this is a massive underestimate due to the vast majority of cases occurring in developing countries where records are not always kept. In 2001, the W.H.O. estimated that yellow fever causes 200,000 illnesses and 30,000 deaths every year in unvaccinated populations.

Origins

This disease was first noted in the Yucatan Peninsula, Mexico, in 1648. It has been the source of several devastating epidemics—during one of Napoleon's campaigns to Haiti in 1802, his troops were attacked by yellow fever and more than half of his army died. Since then, we have worked out that there are two kinds of yellow fever, each spread by a different cycle of infection. Jungle yellow fever infects monkeys in the tropical rain forest, and people are at risk only if they work in the rain forests and are bitten by infected mosquitoes. Because few people live in rain forests, the disease is rare. If, however, you choose to be one of those few, your personal risk of getting it will be high.

Urban yellow fever is more of a threat because more people live in urban areas. The virus is spread by the *Aedes aegypti* mosquito, which thrives in cities, towns, and villages. These mosquitoes breed in the small pools of water that

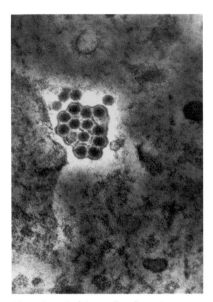

Above Several of these yellow fever virus particles are surrounded by an envelope derived from the host cell membrane. This helps to prevent the host's immune system from recognizing the virus as foreign.

collect in discarded tires, flower pots, oil drums, and open water-storage containers. Thirty-two countries in sub-Saharan Africa experience periodic yet unpredictable outbreaks of urban yellow fever. There are 610 million people living in these countries, of whom the 219 million who live in towns and cites are at particular risk.

Symptoms and effects

Many people only have mild symptoms, but, after a three- to six-day incubation period, others develop high fevers, chills, headaches, vomiting, and backache. Other symptoms may include a red tongue, flushed face, and a reddening of the eyes. After a few days of apparent recovery, they suffer from internal bleeding, and kidney and liver failure. As the liver fails, their skin turns yellow with jaundice—hence the disease's name. If the disease progresses, the victim suffers delerium, seizures and coma.

Region of operation

Outside Africa, yellow fever is part of the health scene in ten South and Central American countries, as well as in several Caribbean islands, with Bolivia, Brazil, Colombia, Ecuador, Peru, and Venezuela considered as the places of greatest risk. People in these countries are currently at more risk than they have been for many years, as the numbers of mosquitoes are rising, and the cities are growing, but the level of vaccination isn't increasing. No one has ever reported a case of yellow fever in Asia. If it did move there, a serious outbreak could result, as the virus's favorite mosquito, *Aedes aegypti*, lives there already.

Historic outbreaks

Yellow fever made an appearance in the United States in the eighteenth, nineteenth, and twentieth centuries. In 1700 and 1793 there were outbreaks in New York and Philadelphia. In 1853, yellow fever moved south to New Orleans, and in 1878 to Memphis. As late as 1905, yellow fever still plagued port cities of the Southern U.S., resulting in 5,000 cases and 1,000 deaths.

Between 1960 and 1962, yellow fever showed its real potential by infecting 100,000 people in Ethiopia, and killing 30,000 of them.

Developments in treatment

There is no specific cure for yellow fever, so treatment is supportive only—rest, fresh air, and plenty of fluids. There is a vaccine, which is a must if you are traveling to infected areas, and gives at least 10 years' immunity from the disease; some countries are attempting to vaccinate their residents. Other ways to avoid contracting the disease include using insecticides, wearing protective clothing, and screening houses, but these are often not enough on their own. Prevention through vaccination is therefore the best route.

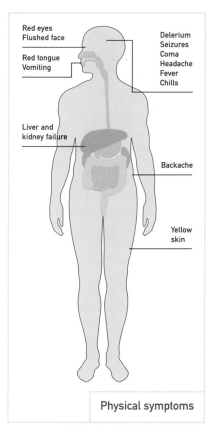

Red eyes
Flushed face

Red tongue
Vomiting

Delerium
Seizures
Coma
Headache
Fever
Chills

Liver and
kidney failure

Backache

Yellow
skin

Physical symptoms

Typhus

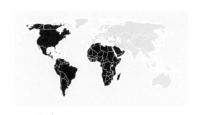

Agent: bacterium, louse (*R. prowazekii*)
and flea (*R. typhi*)
Rickettsia prowazekii and *Rickettsia typhi*
First recorded: 1500s
Region: North and South America,
and Africa

Infectivity	
Severity of illness	
Likelihood of dying if ill	
Bio-weapon threat	

Millions of human lives have been cut short by this louse-borne bacterium, *Rickettsia prowazekii*, and its flea-borne cousin, *Rickettsia typhi*.

Origins

Lice take in the bacteria from the blood of an infected rat or human. Before dying, the louse often bites another human, effectively spitting the bacteria into this person's wound. On top of this, the louse excretes large quantities of bacteria-laden feces that remain infective for weeks. Humans become infected when the dry feces are rubbed into small wounds in the skin, or are inhaled.

Symptoms and effects

These bacteria normally enter the body via an insect bite, then spread quickly in the bloodstream. They break into skin cells, multiply and then break out again, destroying the host cell. With infections of *R. prowazekii*, the initial symptoms are a headache and fever six to 15 days after being bitten. Four to seven days later, a rash appears on the chest, stomach, and back. If the person is lucky, these spots die away over the next couple of days and they recover. The less fortunate go on to develop kidney failure and fall into stupors or comas—the disease gets its name from *typhus*, the Greek word for "stupor." Many of these people will die, but there is a chance of saving them if they are given good medical care. Picking up *R. typhi* from a flea can make someone ill for a month or two, but it rarely kills.

Region of operation

North and South America and Africa are the main zones of operation for *R. prowazekki*, while *R. typhi* lives in tropical and subtropical regions of the world.

Historic outbreaks

This disease can have a devastating effect. In Mexico in 1576, two million died out of a population of nine million, and the probable cause was typhus. History also shows that generals who plan to fight only human foes are prone to run into problems. In 1528, a French army besieging Naples was wiped out by typhus, with 19,000 killed out of a total of 25,000. In 1812, Napoleon set out to invade Russia with around 400,000 soldiers, but during a one-month period over 80,000 were infected with typhus and either died or were too ill to fight.

Developments in treatment

Typhus can be treated by various antibiotics, but many people in poor or devastated areas are not diagnosed, and have no access to the drugs.

Used as a weapon

Typhus will probably never be used as a weapon, but it does show up whenever weapons are used because the breakdown in infrastructure that accompanies conflict creates an ideal breeding ground for lice, fleas, and disease.

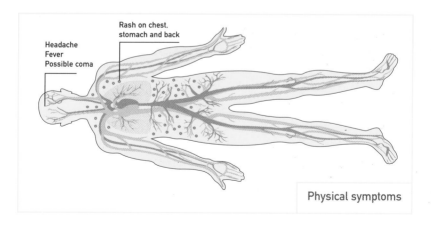

Rash on chest, stomach and back

Headache
Fever
Possible coma

Physical symptoms

Leishmaniasis

Agent: protozoan
Leishmania species and sand fly
First recorded: 1824
Region: tropics and subtropics

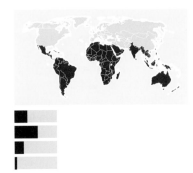

Infectivity
Severity of illness
Likelihood of dying if ill
Bio-weapon threat

There are two versions of leishmaniasis: cutaneous and visceral. With no cure currently available, the single-celled animal that causes both of these diseases is worth avoiding if you can.

Origins

Texts from the South American Inca period in the fifteenth and sixteenth centuries, and then during the Spanish colonization, mention the risk run by seasonal agricultural workers who returned from the Andes with skin ulcers. At the time they called it "valley sickness" or "Andean sickness," but it later became know as "white leprosy" because people were left with scars and deformities that strongly resembled the damage caused by leprosy.

At a similar time, Indian physicians were using the Sanskrit term *kala azar* (meaning "black fever") to describe an ancient disease that we now know as visceral leishmaniasis. In 1756, English medic Alexander Russell examined a Turkish patient and came up with the first medical description of the disease, but it wasn't until 1901 that people started tracking down the micro-organisms that caused it.

Symptoms and effects

In cutaneous leishmaniasis, the person develops one or more skin sores within a few weeks of being bitten by infected sand flies. These may be painful or painless, and may or may not develop a scab. Without treatment, the sores can last from weeks to years, and often develop raised edges and a central crater. In visceral leishmaniasis, sufferers have fevers and lose weight. Their spleen and liver enlarge, and they develop anemia. Untreated, the symptoms gradually get worse over a few months, or possibly a year, and they run a great risk of dying.

Region of operation

Leishmaniasis is found in approximately 90 countries around the world, including those in the tropics, subtropics, and southern Europe. More than 90 percent of visceral leishmaniasis cases occur in Bangladesh, Brazil, India, Nepal, and Sudan. If you want to live in the tropics and still be certain of avoiding it, you could move to Australia, the South Pacific, or South-east Asia, as it hasn't been found there—yet.

Developments in treatment

There are currently no vaccines or drugs that can prevent infections, and there is little available by way of a cure. If you are in an affected area of the world, you need to avoid being bitten by sand flies. Avoid going out at night, and wear clothing that keeps you covered, as well as putting insect repellant on your face, hands, wrists, and ankles. It's easy to underestimate the numbers of bites you get, because sand flies are noiseless fliers and occasional bites might not be noticed. Sleeping under bed nets at night is a good idea, as is having fine mesh at the windows. The mesh does need to be fine, however, as these flies are about one-third of the size of mosquitoes.

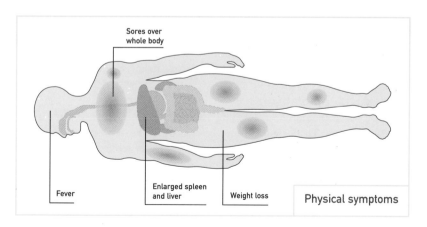

Sores over whole body

Fever

Enlarged spleen and liver

Weight loss

Physical symptoms

Leptospirosis

Agent: bacterium and mammals
Leptospira species
First recorded: 1870
Region: worldwide

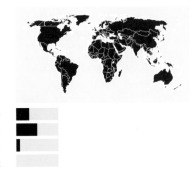

Infectivity	■
Severity of illness	■
Likelihood of dying if ill	▎
Bio-weapon threat	

Becoming infected with any one of the 200 or more species of leptospira bacteria is called "leptospirosis." In a small number of cases, the infection severely damages the organs and causes jaundice.

Symptoms and effects

Not everyone exposed to the disease develops an infection, but if the bacteria take hold and grow, the first symptoms resemble a cold or flu. After an incubation period of four to ten days, people develop fevers, chills, and muscular aches and pains. They lose their appetites, and feel nauseous when lying down. If the symptoms aren't recognized, or no treatment is available, the person's skin starts to bruise. This is caused by blood seeping into the tissues from blood vessels that have been damaged by the bacteria, and results in anemia, which will be accompanied by sore eyes, nose bleeds, and jaundice. The fever lasts for about five days, then the sufferer's health deteriorates to the point that he or she will die without considerable medical support.

Region of operation

Drinking water that has been contaminated by animals is the basic route of infection. Given that the animals may be cattle, pigs, horses, dogs, or rodents, there is every reason to suspect all water running in all streams and rivers—anywhere. The situation is made worse by the fact that many animals—especially rats—can become infected without showing any signs of illness.

    If you work on a farm, go fishing, or enjoy sports like white-water rafting, you will increase your risk of catching the disease. It is well worth mentioning this to your doctor if you ever have an unexplained bout of fever a few days after one of these activities—leptospirosis is not the first thing that will naturally spring to a Western doctor's mind.

Historic outbreaks
Outbreaks are often triggered by a single contaminated source of water that is shared by a large number of people. In June 2004, for example, over 140 children from a Kenyan high school became infected, and six died. A nearby primary school also reported some suspected cases and two more deaths. The schools shared a water source, in which health officials found bacteria.

Developments in treatment
Antibiotics can deal with this infection if it is caught early enough. Vaccinating cattle and domestic animals can help to eradicate the sources of infection.

Potential threat to civilization
Leptospirosis is a problem for humans largely because of our desire to keep and domesticate animals. We keep them on farms and welcome them into our homes as pets. It is a fundamentally important aspect of our civilization, but one that we need to perform with care, as these animal assistants can potentially turn into assassins.

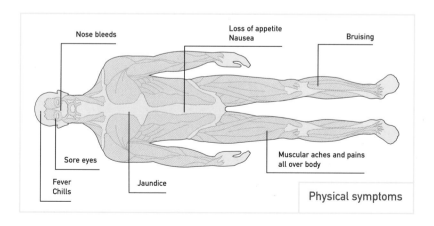

Nose bleeds

Loss of appetite
Nausea

Bruising

Sore eyes

Fever
Chills

Jaundice

Muscular aches and pains
all over body

Physical symptoms

Lyme Disease

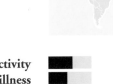

Agent: bacterium and tick
Borrelia burgdorferi
First recorded: 1975
Region: forest areas in the U.S.A.
and U.K.

Infectivity	███
Severity of illness	███
Likelihood of dying if ill	█
Bio-weapon threat	

If you go down to the woods, you need to be prepared for a bite from a tick that could introduce an unwanted bacterium.

Origins
Originally called Lyme's arthritis, this condition was first recorded in 1975 after doctors studied an outbreak of suspected arthritis among young people in the town of Lyme, Connecticut, U.S.A. They soon realized that all of the affected people had recently been bitten by the *Iodes* tick, which lived on deer in the local forests. It turned out that these ticks are themselves infected with *Borrelia burgdorferi*, and studies that looked back at previously unexplained diseases suggest that it has been around in the U.S.A. since at least 1962, and in Europe from the early 1900s. Lyme disease is the most common tick-borne disease in the U.S.A. and Europe, and one of the fastest growing infectious diseases in the U.S.A., where cases have been reported in nearly every state, and with concentrated areas of infection in the northeast, the mid-Atlantic states, Wisconsin, Minnesota, and northern California.

Your chance of picking up the disease depends on which forest you get bitten in. In some forests, two percent of ticks are infected with the disease, while in others the figure rises to 50 percent.

Symptoms and effects
A key characteristic of Lyme disease is a rash called *erythema migrans*. This rash is often described as looking like a bull's-eye on a target, and occurs in about

80 percent of Lyme disease patients. There may be a delay of anything from three to 30 days from the time of the bite to the appearance of this rash. People may also experience symptoms of fatigue, chills, fever, headache, muscle and joint aches, sore throat, sinus infections, and swollen lymph nodes. In some cases, these may be the only symptoms of the infection. In other cases, the symptoms disappear, but the disease still progresses.

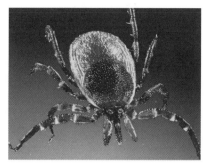

Above The deer tick, or *Ixodes dammini* or *scapularis*, is responsible for transmitting Lyme disease in northern and central U.S.A. The bacteria that cause the disease get passed on when the tick feeds on warm-blooded animals—including humans.

Untreated, the infection will probably spread to other parts of the body. Over the next days or weeks, the person's muscles lose tone on one or both sides of the face and the headaches become severe. As the bacteria move into the tissues around the brain and trigger meningitis, the sufferer's neck stiffens, and shooting pains may start to disturb their sleep. The pain starts to move from joint to joint. Some people will be fortunate, and their immune system will cut in and start destroying the bacteria. However, for approximately 60 percent of infected people who aren't treated, the infection will begin to cause intermittent bouts of arthritis, with severe joint pain and swelling. Around five percent additionally develop shooting pains, numbness or tingling in the hands or feet, and problems with concentration and short-term memory. The later symptoms of Lyme disease can occur months after the initial infection.

If a pregnant woman becomes infected, the bacteria can move to her unborn baby. The result can be serious—the unborn baby may even die.

Historic outbreaks

In the U.S.A. the incidence of Lyme disease has risen steadily: in 1991 there were just under 10,000 recorded cases, but in 2002 nearly 25,000 were reported as having picked up the bug. Whether this is due to increased disease, increased reporting, or both, is difficult to tell—but clearly, people who move into forests for work or play need to take care and look out for rashes.

Developments in treatment

If you spot that a person has Lyme disease early enough and treat them properly with antibiotics, there is every reason to expect a rapid and complete recovery. It is therefore important to spot the first signs. As long as you start early enough, symptoms should disappear quickly once the person starts taking antibiotics, but some can experience months or even years of discomfort once the infection is cleared. Delayed or inadequate treatment may lead to a chronic illness that is disabling and difficult to treat.

However, the symptoms of Lyme disease are such that it can be misdiagnosed as multiple sclerosis, rheumatoid arthritis, fibromyalgia, chronic fatigue syndrome, or a number of other—mainly autoimmune or neurological— diseases. This is a particular problem in areas where Lyme disease is not common and doctors would not therefore immediately think of it. It is thus imperative that anyone who lives, works, or performs leisure pursuits in areas where Lyme disease is likely to be lurking is aware of the possible symptoms and alerts his or her doctor to the possibility of infection.

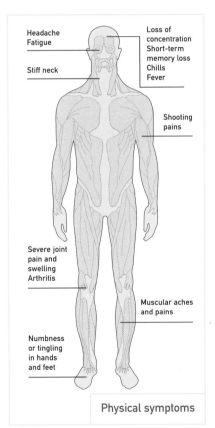

Headache
Fatigue

Stiff neck

Loss of concentration
Short-term memory loss
Chills
Fever

Shooting pains

Severe joint pain and swelling
Arthritis

Muscular aches and pains

Numbness or tingling in hands and feet

Physical symptoms

Dengue Fever

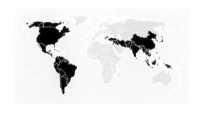

Agent: virus (Family: *Flaviviridae*)
Dengue-1, dengue-2, dengue-3 and
dengue-4 virus
First recorded: 1780
Region: Asia, Americas, Eastern
Mediterranean, South-east Asia, and
Western Pacific

Infectivity	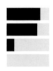
Severity of illness	
Likelihood of dying if ill	
Bio-weapon threat	

The World Health Organization estimates that around 2.5 billion people, some two-fifths of the world's population, are currently at risk from dengue fever. It also believes that up to 50 million people around the world are infected with it each year. It is an important disease.

The disease has two levels of severity. Dengue fever is a mosquito-borne infection that makes you ill, but dengue hemorrhagic fever is a more severe version that may kill you if you do not get good treatment and support.

Origins

An outbreak of fever in Philadelphia in 1780 is the first record of a disease that sounds like dengue fever, but whatever its origins, it is currently on the rise, and by the 1990s was the second most common mosquito-borne disease affecting humans, after malaria. Before 1970, epidemics of dengue hemorrhagic fever had occurred in only nine countries; by 1995, this had increased to almost 40 countries. By 2006, it was fully established in over 100 countries. Consequently, the number of people infected has soared. Between 1995 and 2001, the cases of dengue infection in the Americas doubled from around 300,000 to more than 600,000. This brought the number of people who went on to get full-blown dengue hemorrhagic fever up to over 15,000 a year in that region alone.

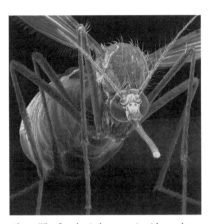

Above The female *Aedes* mosquito (shown here with a swollen abdomen as a result of feeding on blood) is responsible for spreading the viruses that cause dengue fever.

Symptoms and effects

Dengue viruses are transmitted to a person when they are bitten by an infected female *Aedes* mosquito. The viruses circulate in the bloodstream for two to seven days. During this time the person will develop a flu-like illness, with a sudden onset of fever. Infants may get away with just a rash, but older children and adults will be more likely to have a bright red rash, which first appears on the chest but spreads to cover the whole body, accompanied by high temperatures, severe headaches, pain behind the eyes, and muscle and joint pains. The symptoms typically last for between six and seven days, with a smaller peak of fever occurring towards the end of the illness.

About one in 40 people go on to develop dengue hemorrhagic fever. Here, they get a very high temperature, accompanied by abdominal pain, nausea, vomiting, diarrhea, and a lack of appetite. Their liver enlarges, and their body goes into a state of shock. Half of them die within 12 to 24 hours of developing these severe symptoms.

Some people develop much milder symptoms, which can lead to a misdiagnosis of influenza or some other viral infection, especially in cases where the victim doesn't develop a rash. In this way, infected travelers who are not correctly diagnosed at the onset of illness can inadvertently pass on dengue fever when they return to their home countries—and dengue fever is unlikely to be the first thing that springs to mind to doctors in areas that are, on the whole, unaffected by the disease.

Region of operation

To survive, the virus needs mosquitoes, and mosquitoes need water, so the tropics and swampy areas provide ideal conditions for the spread of this disease. In urban areas, the most common breeding zones are not huge swamps, but small pools of water in discarded tires, metal drums, and jars. Domestic water tanks that don't have decent coverings are also superb breeding places. A major way of combating the disease has been to cut old car tires in half and stack them so they can't collect rain water.

Developments in treatment
Tackling this disease is made more complicated by the fact that there are four versions of the virus. It appears that if you vaccinate against two of the viruses, you are more prone to the disease if you meet either of the other two versions. The only option is to develop a vaccine that protects against all four, but such a vaccine is not yet available. Treatment itself consists of rest and support, in particular ensuring that the patient keeps up fluid intake to avoid dehydration.

Potential threat to civilization
Any disease that can kill or cause serious illness, and is infecting increasing numbers of people, needs to be taken very seriously. It will probably not threaten our civilization, but it should make us ask serious questions about the way we plan and build our towns and cities.

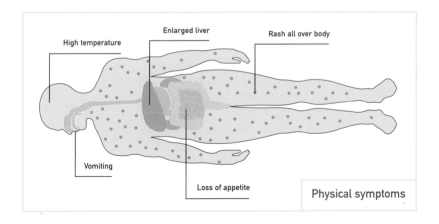

High temperature

Enlarged liver

Rash all over body

Vomiting

Loss of appetite

Physical symptoms

Malaria

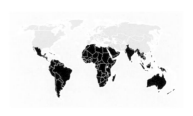

Agent: protozoan and mosquito
Plasmodium falciparum, *Plasmodium vivax*, *Plasmodium ovale*, and *Plasmodium malariae*
First recorded: antiquity
Region: tropics and subtropics

Infectivity	
Severity of illness	
Likelihood of dying if ill	
Bio-weapon threat	

One million people die each year of malaria, a disease that has had a profound impact on human history. Four Nobel Prizes have been awarded to people who have made significant steps in making sense of it, or helping to combat it.

Origins

Malaria means "bad air" and is so-called because the first people who tried to make sense of the disease realized that it was associated with swamps. It isn't the stale air, however, but the insects flying in that air, that are critical.

Symptoms and effects

There are four different types of malaria parasite that share a similar life cycle. When an infected mosquito bites, the parasites move from the mosquito's salivary gland into the person's bloodstream. The parasites are then carried to the liver, where they invade cells and produce many copies of themselves. After a couple of days the cells burst, releasing thousands of new parasites into the bloodstream, and triggering a bout of fever. Other symptoms include shivering, fatigue, and headache; some victims also suffer from nausea, vomiting, and diarrhea.

Once in the bloodstream, these young parasites grow inside red blood cells and turn into either male or female versions of the organism. To develop further in their life cycle, the parasites need to return to a mosquito. When an infected person is bitten again, the mosquito draws up parasites with the blood. Inside the mosquito, the male and female parasites get together and sexually produce the next generation. *P. falciparum* differs from the other three types in that its parasites have a tendency to clump together in the fine capillaries of the brain, which can kill.

Region of operation
The protozoa need mosquitoes, and mosquitoes like it to be hot and wet. Other than that, they are not fussy. This means that they can operate in almost any of the tropical and sub-tropical areas of the world. As mosquitoes are small, they don't tend to fly far, so the disease is more problematic in urban areas where there is always someone else nearby to bite.

Developments in treatment
The main problem with malaria is that no one has come up with a vaccine, and the parasites are good at becoming resistant to drugs. So far, insecticide-treated bed nets are proving to be the most effective weapon.

Potential threat to civilization
Malaria currently threatens many civilizations and communities around the world. The disease prevents many communities developing and leaves them trapped in poverty.

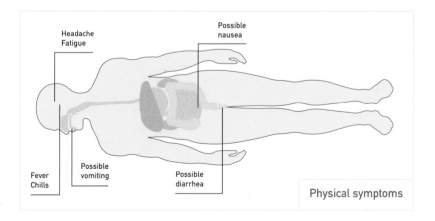

Headache
Fatigue

Possible
nausea

Fever
Chills

Possible
vomiting

Possible
diarrhea

Physical symptoms

Rabies

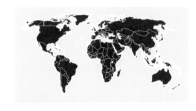

Agent: virus (Family: *Rhabdoviridae*)
Lyssavirus
First recorded: antiquity
Region: worldwide, except for some
islands

Infectivity	
Severity of illness	
Likelihood of dying if ill	
Bio-weapon threat	

Rabies is a bullet-shaped virus that is carried by large carnivorous mammals, such as dogs, cats, and cattle, as well as bats. It gets transferred to people when they get bitten by an infected animal.

Origins

Rabies is derived from the Sanskrit "to do violence," and the disease is one of the oldest documented scourges of humankind. Ancient writers in Mesopotamia, China, Greece, Rome, and India described classic symptoms, although the first complete description was by Italian physician Girolamo Fracastoro in 1546.

Symptoms and effects

The virus normally enters the body through saliva via a bite injury, and attaches to skeletal muscle cells. It multiplies at the wound site, then moves into the nerves. The viruses can then travel to the spinal cord, and eventually to the brain; from here, they use other nerves to move throughout the body. Without treatment, about 80 percent of patients develop a furious form of rabies and wander around in a restless state with a feeling of terror. They develop a severe dislike of water, and die when they can no longer control their muscles enough to breathe. The other 20 percent have a paralytic or dumb form of the disease, in which they simply weaken and die.

One complicating feature of the disease is that the incubation period can be between six days to six or more years. However, if you suspect you have been infected, get help quickly—treatments only work if they are started before symptoms appear.

Region of operation
As with many diseases, there are only vague figures for exactly how many people are infected with it, but rabies is present in most countries around the world. Estimates suggest that between 15,000 and 40,000 people receive treatment for rabies in the U.S.A. In the rest of the world, at least 50,000 people each year don't receive treatment, and consequently die of the disease.

Developments in treatment
Rabies can be treated if caught early enough by injecting the patient with extracts from the blood of animals that have mounted a defense reaction to an attack of rabies. Don't wait before seeking help—if symptoms of the disease have already appeared, it is too late to start treatment, and the disease will almost certainly kill.

Used as a weapon
Threatening to release infected animals in previously rabies-free countries would certainly have a considerable effect as a tool of terror, but in reality it would probably not cause a massive outbreak of the disease among humans.

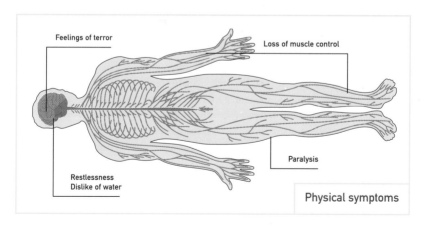

Feelings of terror

Loss of muscle control

Paralysis

Restlessness
Dislike of water

Physical symptoms

Rift Valley Fever

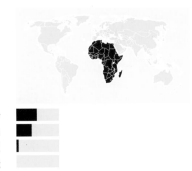

Agent: virus (Family: *Bunyaviridae*)
Rift Valley Fever virus
First recorded: 1930
Region: Africa

Infectivity	██
Severity of illness	██
Likelihood of dying if ill	▎
Bio-weapon threat	

Rift Valley Fever (R.V.F.) mainly affects domestic animals such as cattle, goats, buffalo, sheep, and camels, but it can also affect humans. Epidemics tend to occur after unusually heavy rainfall, when the number of mosquitoes increases.

Origins
In affected areas mosquito eggs are already infected with the virus, so the mosquitoes hatch out fully equipped to infect the livestock on which they feed. Once the livestock is infected, any blood-sucking insect can move the virus to other animals or to humans. Humans can also pick up the disease if they come into contact with the blood or uncooked meat of infected animals.

Symptoms and effects
R.V.F. virus can cause several different sets of symptoms. Some people display no symptoms, while others have a mild fever and short-term problems with their livers. In others, however, the disease causes blood vessels to break down, leading to hemorrhages. If the virus sets up an infection in the brain, victims can have seizures. People who do become ill usually experience fever, general weakness, back pain, dizziness, and extreme weight loss at the onset of the illness. Typically, patients recover within two days to one week. About two percent are left with some damage to their eyes, and one percent die.

Region of operation
The virus is usually found in Eastern and Southern Africa, particularly in areas where sheep and cattle are raised, as well as sub-Saharan Africa and Madagascar.

Historic outbreaks

One way of killing humans is to take away their livestock, so the death of 100,000 sheep in Kenya in 1950–51 due to Rift Valley fever was a distinct human as well as agricultural tragedy. In 1987, the virus triggered its first epidemic in West Africa. The outbreak occurred in an area where people were working on the Senegal River Project, flooding large parts of the lower Senegal River area. This altered the local interactions between animals and humans, and produced a situation where Rift Valley fever could take hold. A few years later, in September 2000, Saudi Arabia and Yemen reported that they had some cases of the disease, but these are the only times that Rift Valley fever has occurred outside Africa.

Developments in treatment

As with many diseases that only affect people in the developing world, there is little financial incentive to develop treatments. On top of this, the disease is caused by a virus, and medical science has not been particularly successful at combating these. Add the two together and it is no surprise that there is no affordable treatment yet—and none is going to appear any time soon.

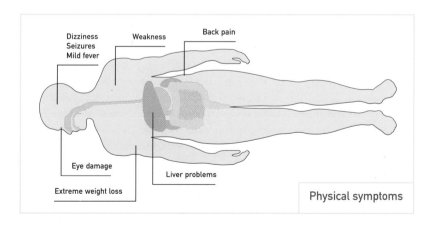

Dizziness
Seizures
Mild fever

Weakness

Back pain

Eye damage

Liver problems

Extreme weight loss

Physical symptoms

West Nile Virus

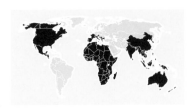

Agent: virus
West Nile virus
First recorded: 1937
Region: Southern Europe, Africa, Central and South Asia, Oceania, and North America

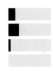

Infectivity	■
Severity of illness	■
Likelihood of dying if ill	|
Bio-weapon threat	

The main way this virus gets around is on board birds, who cover large distances on their annual migrations; it then uses mosquitoes to jump to other animals.

Origins
West Nile virus was first isolated in 1937 in the West Nile district of Uganda, but is now known to have a hold in most of the world where mosquitoes live.

Symptoms and effects
The symptoms vary widely from person to person. Around eight out of 10 infected people will not show any symptoms at all. The rest will get symptoms such as mild fever, headache, body aches, nausea, vomiting, and sometimes swollen lymph glands, or a skin rash on the chest, stomach, and back. When symptoms occur, they normally start between three and 14 days after being bitten by an infected mosquito, and can last for a few days or for several weeks.

About one in 150 infected people have more severe symptoms, including a high fever, headache, neck stiffness, stupor, disorientation, coma, tremors, vision loss, convulsions, muscle weakness, numbness, and paralysis. These symptoms can last for several weeks, and there may even be permanent brain damage.

Region of operation
One of the main areas affected by this virus is Israel, but the largest outbreak triggered 3,000 cases of the disease in South Africa in 1974.

Historic outbreaks

In the late summer of 1999, West Nile virus showed up on the East coast of North America, near New York. There was widespread anxiety, coupled with mass use of insecticides—so much so that many of the shellfish in local estuaries were killed off as the chemicals ran off into the ocean. Within a few months, 61 people had become infected and seven had died. Over the next few years, the virus became established in 11 states along the Eastern coast, and will almost inevitably move into other areas of the continent.

Developments in treatment

There is no treatment other than giving people good medical support and hoping that their body fights the disease itself. The best way to fight it is not to get it—and the best way to do this is to get rid of pools of standing water that give home to mosquitoes.

Used as a weapon

Some conspiracy theorists suggest that West Nile virus was deliberately introduced into the United States by a terror organization. This is theoretically possible, but seems unlikely. You would need to import a vast number of infected mosquitoes to be sure of triggering an epidemic; if you wanted to cause trouble there are other more likely candidates to choose before West Nile virus.

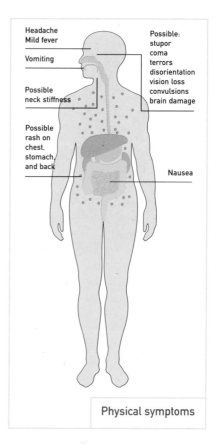

Headache
Mild fever

Vomiting

Possible
neck stiffness

Possible
rash on
chest,
stomach,
and back

Possible:
stupor
coma
terrors
disorientation
vision loss
convulsions
brain damage

Nausea

Physical symptoms

Nipah Virus

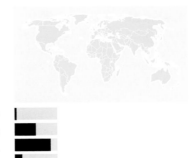

Agent: virus (Family: *Paramyxoviridae*)
Nipah virus
First recorded: 1999
Region: Malaysia

Infectivity	
Severity of illness	
Likelihood of dying if ill	
Bio-weapon threat	

Has it always existed but we've only just noticed, or is it the result of a large-scale mutation from a previous virus? The question is not simple to answer, because Nipah virus entered medical literature only in 1999. The virus is named for the place where it was found—Nipah in Malaysia.

Origins
One the whole, this virus lives in animals, but it can jump to humans—and it is not nice.

Symptoms and effects
Many people seem to become infected by this virus without producing symptoms—quite how many is difficult to tell with a virus that has been so recently discovered. For those that do have symptoms, they start after an incubation period of between four and 18 days. Initially, the person develops flu-like symptoms, with high fever and muscle pains. Some then get better, but others develop an inflammation of the brain, become drowsy and disorientated, and have convulsions. Around half these people die.

Region of operation
At the moment, Nipah virus seems to be confined to Malaysia, Bangladesh, and Singapore. Initial reports suggest that, when it is not at work in humans, it survives in a particular species of bat that lives in those parts. However, the virus seems to jump to humans via pigs and cattle. If it starts residing in large numbers of these animals, it could become a critically important disease.

Historic outbreaks

The first known outbreak occurred between September 1998 and May 1999 and caused 265 people in Malaysia to develop brain inflammation, more than 100 of whom died. Most of the people affected were pig farmers. At the same time, 11 cases and one death occurred in Singapore. All of these were people who worked in an abattoir that slaughtered pigs imported from affected areas of Malaysia. The outbreak was contained by the mass culling of more than one million pigs, and since then, no other outbreaks of Nipah virus have been reported in Malaysia. It has showed up elsewhere, though. Between January and February 2004, 46 people in Bangladesh became infected with Nipah virus, and 35 of them died.

Developments in treatment

Given that we have no treatment for many viral diseases that we have known about for decades, no one should be surprised that we have no treatment for such a recently discovered virus.

Used as a weapon

If you could capture and control a disease that human populations have never encountered before, you would have a huge terror threat. The problem with this is that, if you unleashed it, you would probably kill as many friends as foes.

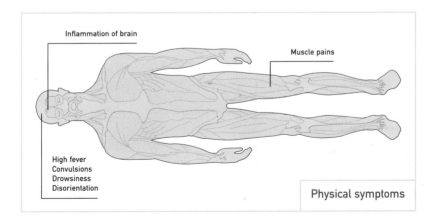

Inflammation of brain

Muscle pains

High fever
Convulsions
Drowsiness
Disorientation

Physical symptoms

Rocky Mountain Spotted Fever

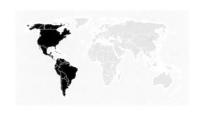

Agent: bacterium
Rickettsia rickettsii
First recorded: 1896
Region: North and South Americas

Infectivity
Severity of illness
Likelihood of dying if ill
Bio-weapon threat

This is another disease that should make you think twice before wandering into the woods wearing short trousers and a T-shirt. This time, you need to keep covered to avoid a tick-borne bacterial disease that, in the pre-antibiotic world, was frequently fatal.

Origins

Originally called "black measles," the infective bacteria responsible for what is now known as Rocky Mountain Spotted Fever was first discovered in the Snake River Valley of Idaho in 1896. It was initially studied by American medic Howard T. Ricketts—hence the bacterium's name.

Symptoms and effects

Rickettsia rickettsii grow inside the cells of small and medium-sized blood vessels within its victim. They multiply and destroy the cells, causing the blood vessels to become leaky and leading to the development of black spots all over the person's body. Early symptoms are much like so many other diseases—feeling a bit weak with a fever, nausea, vomiting, and headache. After around a week, however, a rash starts to develop in most, though not all, infected people.

If the infection is not hit hard and early with antibiotics, the victim may need to be hospitalized. He or she could end up with long-term damage to the internal organs and partial paralysis. The breakdown in circulation leaves some people with gangrene in their fingers and toes, which may need amputating.

Region of operation

The bacterium lives inside ticks that inhabit woodlands in the Americas, and causes between 250 and 1,200 cases of the disease in the U.S.A. each year. The vast majority of these occur between March and August—the time when the ticks are most active, and people are more likely to go trekking in the woods.

Developments in treatment

Antibiotics have greatly increased the chance of surviving this disease, but they do need to be started early. This can mean starting to take a course of the drugs before the disease has been confirmed.

Used as a weapon

In many tick-borne diseases the tick acts as a vector, carrying the disease from the infected animal to the human. This would be a difficult model to use as a weapon. In the case of Rocky Mountain Spotted Fever, however, the tick not only transports the disease, but is also the natural reservoir of the disease. Therefore, it would theoretically be easier to deliberately introduce this to an area, if you were so inclined. Because most people live in urban areas, however, it would have little overall impact in terms of numbers, but releasing it could grab headlines for some terror group.

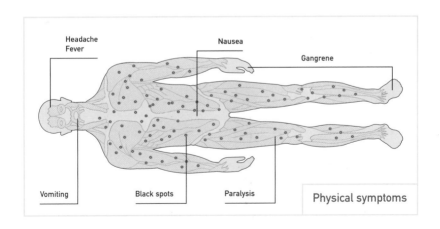

Headache
Fever

Nausea

Gangrene

Vomiting

Black spots

Paralysis

Physical symptoms

Lassa Fever

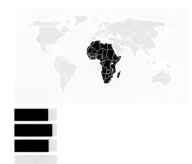

Agent: virus (Family: *Arenaviridae*)
Lassa virus
First recorded: 1969
Region: Western Africa

Infectivity	
Severity of illness	
Likelihood of dying if ill	
Bio-weapon threat	

A disease that is highly infectious and very likely to kill if you get it is the stuff of nightmares, but Lassa fever has another twist—no one knows where it comes from. The best guess is that a type of small rodent known as the multimammate rat carries the virus and passes it to humans in its urine and feces.

Origins
Lassa virus was first identified in 1969 in a blood sample taken from a nurse in Jos, Nigeria. She turned out to be fourth in a line of victims that had started with a young woman who sought medical help for a bacterial blood infection as a result of having an abortion. The virus turned out to be one of a small group of highly dangerous infectious agents that includes Ebola and Marburg.

Symptoms and effects
This disease has a relatively slow start. It seems to wait for between one and three weeks before triggering symptoms, then gradually a fever and headache set in. Joint pain, sore throats, and a non-productive cough follow soon after, and in severe cases people start to vomit and have diarrhea. As their blood and blood vessels become damaged, their faces and necks become puffy and swollen.

If you are going to survive, you will recover within one to three weeks. If not, more symptoms develop, including bleeding gums and nose, low blood pressure, and an inability to produce urine. Around one-quarter of people go permanently deaf, and some have seizures. One in eight patients who have to go to hospital do not come out alive. One in five pregnant women who get the disease die and nine out of 10 pregnant women who survive lose their baby.

Region of operation

The disease seems to be restricted to areas of the world inhabited by the multimammate rat, which is found only in Western Africa. At greatest risk are people who live in rural areas where sanitation is poor or accommodation is over-crowded. Health-care workers are at particular risk if they don't use proper barrier nursing and infection-control practices.

Historic outbreaks

This disease tends to hide away for a bit, then break out and infect a number of people at once. Between January 1 and April 24, 2004, 95 young people were admitted to a hospital in Sierra Leone with Lassa fever. Three-quarters of these had spent some time over the previous weeks on the pediatric ward of the same hospital. Most probably, an individual patient had brought the disease in, and it was then spread either by direct contact, or by medical staff not sterilizing equipment such as re-usable needles. Almost three-quarters of the patients died.

Developments in treatment

It just so happens that the antiviral drug ribavirin is an effective treatment for Lassa fever, but only if given early enough in the course of clinical illness—and then it is available only if you can afford it.

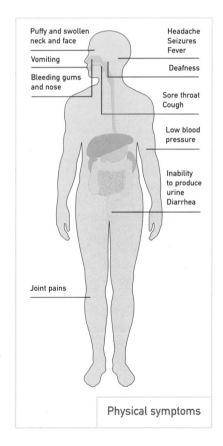

Puffy and swollen neck and face

Vomiting

Bleeding gums and nose

Headache
Seizures
Fever

Deafness

Sore throat
Cough

Low blood pressure

Inability to produce urine
Diarrhea

Joint pains

Physical symptoms

Sources

Books
Albert, Bruce, *Essential Cell Biology* (Garland Science: New York, 2003)
Smith, Tony, *British Medical Association Complete Family Health Encyclopaedia* (Dorling Kindersley: London, 1995)

Websites
www.about-ecoli.com
www.aboutibs.org
www.about-salmonella.com
www.always-health.com
www.amm.co.uk
www.astdhpphe.org
www.avert.org
www.biomedcentral.com/news
www.bt.cdc.gov
www.cdc.gov
www.cdiffsupport.com
www.cjd.ed.ac.uk
www.emedicine.com
www.healthlink.mcw.edu
www.healthywomen.org
www.helico.com
www.herpes-coldsores.com
www.homehealth-uk.com
www.itg.be
www.kidshealth.org
www.leprosymission.org
www.mdheal.org
www.medinfo.co.uk
www.nathnac.org
www.nature.com

www.netdoctor.co.uk
news.bbc.co.uk
www.newscientist.com
www.niaid.nih.gov
www.nobelprize.org
www.pandemicflu.gov
www.patient.co.uk
www.plospathogens.org
www.rotavirusvaccine.org
www.scidev.net
www.scienceinafrica.co.za
www.stanford.edu/group/virus/1999/
   rahul23/timeline.html
www.textbookofbacteriology.net
www.themiddleages.net
www.tudorplace.com.ar
www.uspharmacist.com
www.who.int/wer

Glossary

antibiotic: a drug that kills or slows the growth of bacteria.

antibody: a protein used by the immune system to identify foreign objects like bacteria and viruses.

antitoxin: an antibody with the ability to neutralize a specific toxin.

antiviral: a drug that works against viruses.

bacteriophage: a virus that destroys bacteria.

bacterium: a microscopic single-celled organism found in soil, water, and food, or in humans and animals. Most do no harm, but a few cause serious diseases.

biotype: a group of organisms that share the same genotype.

bubo: an inflamed swelling of the lymph glands, especially in the groin or armpit.

cell: the smallest unit of living matter in animals or plants.

chancre: a painless ulcer formed during the primary stage of syphilis.

chronic infection: a long-lasting infection, or with symptoms that are apt to recur.

circulatory system: the system that moves substances to and from cells; the main components are the heart, the blood, and the blood vessels.

contagion: the passing of a disease by touching an infected person.

cutaneous: affecting the skin.

digestive system: the system of organs that takes in food, digests it to extract energy and nutrients, and expels the remaining waste.

DNA: deoxyribonucleic acid—a helically twisting molecule that holds biological genetic instructions in cells and many viruses.

ecosystem: a community of organisms and its environment.

endemic: refers to a disease that is constantly present in a particular locality or people.

epidemic: an outbreak of a disease that attacks many people in a community at the same time.

gene: a single biological instruction within a molecule of DNA.

genetic code: the full set of genetic instructions held within a single cell.

hemmorhage: an abnormal flow of blood from the heart, arteries, veins, or capillaries.

host: an animal or plant on which another is parasitic.

immune system: the system that protects the body from infection.

immunity: having sufficient biological defenses to avoid infection.

immunosuppressants: drugs that minimize the body's natural reaction to foreign substances; they are for example used to prevent bodies rejecting transplanted organs.

incubation period: the period between infection and the development of symptoms of a disease.

instruction set: a set of genetic instructions.

jump change: a sizable change in one step.

lymph nodes: components of the lymphatic system that act as filters to collect and destroy bacteria and viruses.

lymphatic system: the body system that transports lymph fluid from tissues to the circulatory system. It is a major component of the immune system.

metastasis: the spread of cancer from its primary site to other places in the body.

nephrology: the scientific study of the kidneys.

nervous system: the biological system that coordinates the activity of the muscles, monitors the organs, sends information to the brain from the sensory receptors, processes that information, and initiates actions.

pandemic: an outbreak of a disease that affects a whole country or the whole world.

parasite: an animal or plant that exists at the expense of another organism.

pasteurization: a process that uses heat to destroy dangerous organisms in food, but avoids damaging the food.

prion: an infectious protein particle associated with a rare group of brain and nervous system diseases.

protozoa: microscopic single-celled organisms.

resistance: the body's power to withstand a disease, or an organism's ability to avoid the effects of a drug.

respiratory system: the biological system that enables an animal to take in oxygen and get rid of carbon dioxide. In humans, it consists of the airways, the lungs, and the respiratory muscles that force air in and out of the chest.

sputum: a mixture of saliva and mucus.

strain: a variant of a disease, bacterium, or virus.

toxin: a poisonous compound causing a particular disease.

ulcer: an open sore on the outer or inner surface of the body, often accompanied by pus or another discharge.

vaccine: an agent that makes people immune to a disease so that they are protected from future infections of the virus or bacteria.

virus: a microscopic particle that can infect the cells of a biological organism, consisting of genetic material contained within a protective protein shell. They can only reproduce inside a host cell.

visceral: relating to the "viscera," or the internal organs.

Index